MEDITERRANEAN DIET

FOR BEGINNERS

# MEDITERRANEAN
# LOVERS DIET

*A Delicious Yet Quick &*
*Easy Plant Based Diet*
*Cookbook For Beginners*

*(Simple Recipes and Ingredients to Start)*

## ANDERSON ARIAS

# Table of Contents

# PART I

# Chapter 1: Identifying the Mediterranean Diet

We know that certain diets are associated with better health—this is a simple fact of life. We've seen that entire groups of people live longer based on where they live, and to some degree, a good deal of that has to come from somewhere—it has to come from something like diet or environment. In this case, the diet of the people living in the Mediterranean has been found to be incredibly healthy for people—it has been shown that people who are able to enjoy this diet, who are able to eat fresh food by the sea and enjoy the benefits that it has, are able to be far healthier than those who don't have it. That is great for them—but what is their secret?

It turns out, it's all in the lifestyle. The Mediterranean lifestyle, food, and all, is incredibly healthy for you. Studies have shown that people living in Mediterranean countries such as Greece and Italy have been found to have far less risk of death from coronary disease. Their secret is in the diet. Their diet has been shown to reduce the risk of cardiovascular disease, meaning that it is incredibly healthy, beneficial, and something that the vast majority of people in the world could definitely benefit from.

The Mediterranean diet is recommended by doctors and the World Health Organization as being not only healthy but also sustainable, meaning that it is something that is highly recommended, even by the experts. If you've found that you've struggled with weight loss, heart disease, managing your blood pressure, or anything similar to those problems, then the Mediterranean diet is for you. When you follow this diet, you are able to bring health back to your life and enjoy the foods while doing so. It's perfect if you want to be able to enjoy your diet without having to worry about the impacts that it will have on you.

## Defining the Mediterranean Lifestyle

The Mediterranean diet is quite simple. It involves eating traditional foods based on one's location. Typically, in the Mediterranean, that is a diet that is rich in veggies, fruits, whole grains, beans, and features olive oil as the fat of choice. Typically, it involves elements beyond just eating as well. While it is important to have healthy food, it is equally important to recognize that the diet encompasses the lifestyle as well. In particular, you can expect to see a few other rules come into play.

In particular, the Mediterranean diet is unique in the sense that it encourages a glass of red wine every now and then. In fact, the diet is associated with moderate drinking, enjoying red wine several times per week, always responsibly, and in contexts that will be beneficial to the drinker. If you want to be able to enjoy the Mediterranean diet and you are pregnant, or against drinking, you can do that, too—but traditionally, the red wine is included and even encouraged in moderation thanks to the antioxidants within it.

Additionally, on the Mediterranean diet, it is common to share meals with friends and family. This is essential—eating is more than just filling the body, it is nurturing the mind and relationships as well. This also comes with the added benefit of also being able to slow down eating—when you are eating the foods on this diet, you will discover that ultimately, you eat less when you're busy having a riveting conversation with someone. The fact that you are slowed down with your eating means that you will fill up sooner and realize that you didn't have to actually eat the food that you did. This means that you eat less and are, therefore managing your portions better as a result.

Finally, the Mediterranean diet focuses on physical activity. Traditionally, you would have had to go out to get the foods that you would eat each day, and that would mean that you'd need to get up, fish, garden, farm, or otherwise prepare your food. Eating locally is still a major component of this diet, as is getting up and being active. You need at least 30 minutes of activity, moderate or mild, per day. Even just walking for half an hour is better than nothing!

## The Rules of the Mediterranean Diet

To eat the Mediterranean way, there are a few key factors that can guide you. If you know what you are doing, you can eat well without having to sacrifice flavor for health, and that matters immensely. When you look at the Mediterranean diet closely, you see that there are several tips that will help you to recognize what you need to do to stick to your diet.

### Eating fruits and veggies

First, make sure that the bulk of your calories come from fruits and vegetables. You should be eating between 7 and 10 servings of fresh fruits and vegetables every single day—meaning that the bulk of your calories will come from there.

Try to stick to locally grown foods that are fresh and in-season—they will have the highest nutritional value.


Reach for the whole grains

Yes, pasta is a major part of the diet in the Mediterranean, and you don't have to give that up entirely—but make sure that any grains that you are enjoying are whole-wheat. This allows you to enjoy foods that are high in fiber and are able to be digested differently than when you use refined carbs instead. While the refined carbs may give you instantaneous energy, they are also not nearly as good for you as whole wheat.


Using healthy fats

When it comes to flavoring or cooking your foods, you need to reach for the healthy fats first. This means choosing out foods that are cooked with olive oil instead of butter or dipping food in olive oil instead of butter. Olive oil, despite being a fat, has not been found to lead to weight gain when used in moderation. It is an incredibly healthy substitute for butter that is loaded up with all sorts of beneficial, heart-healthy antioxidants that will help your cardiovascular system.


Aim for seafood

When it comes to protein, fish, especially fresh fish, is the best choice. Fish should be consumed at least twice per week, and it should be fresh rather than frozen whenever possible. In particular, it is commonly recommended that you reach for salmon or trout, or other fatty fish because the omega-3 fatty acids within them are incredibly healthy for you, and they will serve you well. Even better, if you grill your fish, you have little cleanup.

Reduce red meat

In addition to adding more seafood to your diet, you need to cut out the red meat. The red meats in your diet are no good for you—they have been linked to inflammation that can make it harder for your cardiovascular system.

Enjoy dairy in moderation

When you are on this diet, dairy is not out of the picture entirely. While you should avoid butter, for the most part, it is a good idea for you to enjoy some low-fat Greek yogurt on occasion and add in some cheese to your diet. It is a good thing for you to enjoy these foods to ensure that you have plenty of calcium to keep your body strong.

Spices, not salt

Perhaps one of the most profound differences between most other diets and the Mediterranean diet is the lack of salt. The Mediterranean diet reaches for herbs and spices before adding in salt, meaning that you will be consuming less of it over time. Even better, you will grow to love your new foods without needing salt.

# Chapter 2: Savory Mediterranean Meals

Mediterranean Feta Mac and Cheese

Ingredients

- Egg (1, beaten)
- Feta cheese (8 oz., crumbles)
- Macaroni (0.5 lb., whole-wheat)
- Olive oil (3 Tbsp.)
- Salt and pepper to taste
- Sour cream (8 oz.)

Instructions

1. Cook pasta to instructions to create al dente pasta. Drain and place pasta into baking dish. Toss in feta and oil and mix well.
2. Combine your egg and sour cream with salt and pepper. Then mix well and toss over macaroni. Combine and bake at 350F for 30 minutes.

Chickpea Stew

Ingredients

- Bay leaf (1)
- Dry chickpeas (1 c., soaked overnight and peeled)
- Garlic (1 clove, cut in half)
- Lemon to serve

- Olive oil (0.25 c.)
- Onion (1, diced)
- Salt and pepper to taste

Instructions

1. Cover chickpeas in pot with just enough water to cover them and wait to boil. Then rinse and set into clean pot. Toss in all other ingredients but the lemon with just enough water to cover nearly one inch above the beans. Simmer for 2-3 hours and serve with lemons.

Savory Mediterranean Breakfast Muffins

Ingredients

*Dry ingredients*

- Baking powder (1.5 tsp)
- Baking soda (o.5 tsp)
- Flour (2 c.)
- Salt (0.5 tsp)

*Wet ingredients*

- Egg (1 large)
- Garlic (1 clove, minced)
- Milk (1 c.)
- Sour cream (0.25 c.)
- Vegetable oil (0.25 c.)

*Fillings*

- Cheddar cheese (2 c., shredded)
- Feta (2.5 oz., crumbled)
- Green olives (diced, 0.5 c.)
- Green onions (0.5 c., chopped)
- Roasted red peppers (0.5 c., chopped)
- Sun dried tomatoes (diced, 0.5 c.)

Instructions

1. Combine dry ingredients in a bowl. Mix wet ingredients in separate bowl. Combine the two together and mix.
2. Toss in fillings in as few stirs as possible.
3. Place in greased or lined muffin pan, dividing to all 12 recesses.
4. Bake for 25 minutes until golden-brown and crusty at 350F.
5. Cool for 10 minutes and serve warm.

Mediterranean Breakfast Bake

Ingredients

- Artichoke hearts (14-oz. can, drained)
- Bread (6 slices whole-wheat, chopped)
- Eggs (8)
- Feta cheese (0.5 c.)
- Italian sausage (turkey or chicken—1 lb., casings removed)
- Milk (1 c.)
- Olive oil (2 Tbsp., divided)

- Onion (1, chopped)
- Spinach (5 oz.)
- Sun dried tomato (1 c., chopped)

Instructions

1. Warm 1 Tbsp. of your olive oil on moderately high heat. Cook sausage for 8 minutes until it has browned, breaking it up as it cooks. Place it in a dish when it is done.
2. Toss in additional oil, then cook onion until soft, roughly 5 minutes. Toss in spinach until wilting (1 minute).
3. Combine eggs and mix in milk, bread, tomatoes, cheese, artichokes, sausage, and finally, the spinach mix.
4. Place everything in a 2.5 quart baking dish. Let sit for an hour in fridge, or leave overnight.
5. Let casserole sit for 30 minutes after removing from fridge. Then, bake for 45 minutes at 350F until brown. Let rest 10 minutes, then serve.

## Mediterranean Pastry Pinwheels

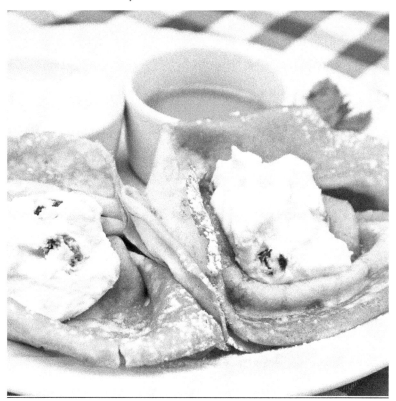

Ingredients

- Cream cheese (8-ounce package, softened)
- Pesto (0.25 c.)
- Provolone cheese (0.75 c.)
- Sun-dried tomatoes (0.5 c., chopped)
- Ripe olives (0.5 c., chopped)

Instructions

1. Unroll pastry and trim it up to create 10-inch square.

2. Mix together your cream cheese and pesto until well-combined. Then, mix in other ingredients until combined. Place mixture in even layer across pastry, up to 0.5-inch of edges. Roll and freeze for 30 minutes.
3. Cut whole roll into 16 pieces.
4. Bake at 400F until golden, roughly 15 minutes. Serve.

# Chapter 3: Sweet Treats on the Mediterranean Diet

Greek Yogurt Parfait

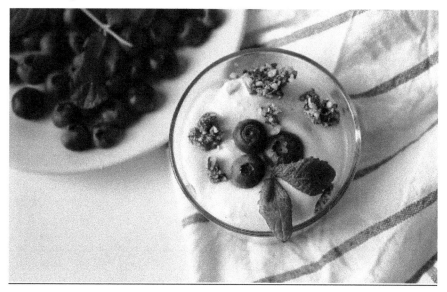

Ingredients

- Almond butter (2 Tbsp.)
- Fresh fruit (1 Tbsp.)
- Greek Yogurt (1 c.)

Instructions

1. Mix together yogurt and 1 Tbsp. of almond butter and put in a bowl. Top with fruit.
2. Warm remaining butter in microwave for 10 minutes, then drizzle atop yogurt. Serve. You can add different toppings to change up the flavor as well.

# Overnight Oats

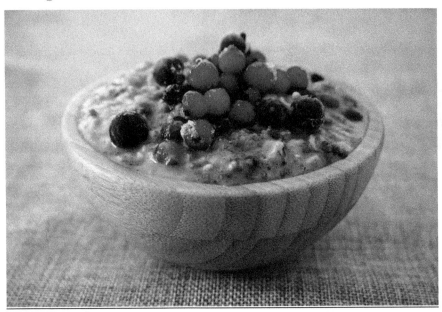

## Ingredients

- Chia seeds (1 Tbsp.)
- Greek yogurt (0.25 c.)
- Honey (1 Tbsp.)
- Milk of choice (0.5 c.)
- Old fashioned whole oats (0.5 c.)
- Vanilla extract (0.25 tsp)

## Instructions

1. Mix all ingredients into a glass container and leave in fridge for at least 2 hours but preferably overnight. Serve with berries of choice or other desired toppings.

## Apple Whipped Yogurt

Ingredients

- Greek yogurt (1 c.)
- Heavy cream (0.5 c.)
- Honey (1 Tbsp.)
- Unsalted butter (2 Tbsp.)
- Apples (2, cored and chopped into small bits)
- Sugar (2 Tbsp.)
- Cinnamon (1/8 tsp)
- Walnut halves (0.25 c., chopped)

Instructions

1. Using a hand mixer, mix together yogurt, honey, and honey until it creates peaks.
2. Heat up your butter in a skillet over a moderate temperature. Cook apples and 1 Tbsp. sugar in pan. Stir and cook for 6-8 minutes until soft. Then, top with the rest of sugar and cinnamon, stirring and cooking an additional 3 minutes. Take it off of the burner and let it rest for 5 minutes.
3. Serve with whipped yogurt in bowl topped with apple, then sprinkle on walnuts.

# Chapter 4: Gourmet Meals on the Mediterranean Diet

Garlic-Roasted Salmon and Brussels Sprouts

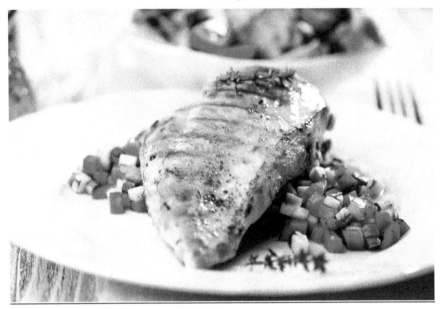

Ingredients

- Brussels sprouts (6 c., trimmed and halved)
- Chardonnay (0.75 c.)
- Garlic cloves (14 large)
- Olive oil (0.25 c.)
- Oregano (2 Tbsp., fresh)
- Pepper (0.75 tsp)
- Salmon fillet (2 lbs., skin-off—cut in 6 pieces)
- Salt (1 tsp)
- Lemon wedges to serve

Instructions

1. Take two cloves of garlic and mince, combining them with oil, 1 Tbsp. of oregano, half of the salt and 1/3 of the pepper. Cut remaining cloves of garlic in halves and toss them with the sprouts. Take 3 Tbsp. of your garlic oil and toss it with the sprouts in roasting pan. Roast for 15 minutes at 450F.

2. Add wine to the remainder of the oil mixture. Then, remove it from the pan, stir veggies, and place salmon atop it all. Pour the wine mix atop it and season with remaining oregano and salt and pepper. Bake 5-10 minutes until salmon is done. Serve alongside the wedged lemon.

Walnut Crusted Salmon with Rosemary

Ingredients

- Dijon mustard (2 tsp)
- Garlic (1 clove, minced)
- Honey (0.5 tsp)
- Kosher salt (0.5 tsp)
- Lemon juice (1 tsp)
- Lemon zest (0.25 tsp.)
- Olive oil (1 tsp)
- Olive oil spray
- Panko (3 Tbsp.)
- Red pepper (0.25 tsp)
- Rosemary (1 tsp, chopped)

- Salmon (1 pound, skin removed)
- Walnuts (3 Tbsp., finely chopped)
- Parsley and lemon to garnish

Instructions

1. Mix together the mustard, lemon zest and juice, honey, salt and red pepper, and rosemary. In a separate dish, combine the panko with oil and walnuts.
2. Spread mustard across salmon and top with panko mixture. Spray fillets with cooking spray.
3. Cook until fish begins to flake at 425F, roughly 8-10 minutes. Serve with lemon and parsley.

## Spaghetti and Clams

Ingredients

- Clams (6.5 lbs.)
- Olive oil (6 Tbsp.)
- White wine (0.5 c.)
- Garlic (3 cloves, sliced)
- Chiles (3, small and crumbled)
- Spaghetti (1 lb.)
- Parsley (3 Tbsp., chopped)
- Salt and pepper to personal preference

Instructions

1. Prepare clams, soaking in clean water and brushing to remove all sand.

2. Warm 2 Tbsp. of oil in large pot. Then, toss in 0.25 c. wine, 1 of the cloves of garlic, and 1 chile. Cook half of the plans at high heat with regular shaking until clams are opened. Remove opened clams and their juices to a larger bowl. Repeat process with second half of clams. Discard any that do not open.

3. Prepare pasta according to packaging to create al dente pasta. Reserve 1 c. pasta water.

4. Warm remainder of oil (2 Tbsp.) in pot over moderate heat, tossing in remainder of garlic and chile. Cook until fragrant, then place all clams and their juices into the pot, tossing to coat well. Then, toss in pasta, mixing well to combine. If necessary, add in cooking liquid. Serve and season with salt/pepper to personal preference with parsley atop.

Braised Lamb and Fennel

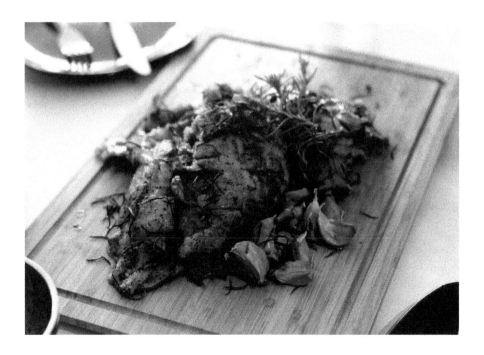

Ingredients

- Bay leaves (2)
- Chicken broth (3 c.)
- Cinnamon stick (1)
- Fennel (1 bulb, chopped)
- Garlic head (chopped in half)
- Lamb shoulder (3 lbs., cut into 8 pieces)
- Olive oil (2 Tbsp.)
- Onion (1, chopped
- Orange (1 with peel, cut into wedges)
- White wine (1 c.)
- Whole peeled tomatoes (14.5 oz. can)

Instructions

1. Dry lamb and season with salt and pepper to taste. Warm oil inside a Dutch oven, and sear lamb on all sides, roughly 6 minutes each side. Move lamb to plate.
2. Place fennel, garlic, and onion in the pot and cook, until browning, roughly 8 minutes. Mix in wine and boil, deglazing the pan. Reduce heat and simmer until it has reduced 50%.
3. Toss in orange, bay leaves, tomatoes, broth, and cinnamon, plus the lamb. Simmer, then cover pot and transfer to oven set to 325F. braise for 1.5-2 hours. Remove lamb and place on clean plate.
4. Strain liquid left in pot, then return it to the pot to boil until thick, roughly 30 minutes.
5. Return lamb to pot to warm. Serve.

## Mediterranean Cod

### Ingredients

- Black olives (0.66 c., sliced)
- Cod (4 fillets, skinless)
- Fennel seeds (1 tsp)
- Lemon (1, sliced)
- Lemon (juice of ½ lemon)
- Olive oil (6 Tbsp.)
- Onion (1, sliced)
- Parsley (1 Tbsp., chopped)
- Salt and pepper to personal preference
- Tomatoes (0.66 c., diced)

### Instructions

1. Warm olive oil at a moderate temperature, sautéing the onion with a pinch of salt until translucent, roughly 10 minutes.
2. Mix in tomato and olives, tossing in the juice as well. Allow it to simmer gently for roughly 5 minutes. Toss in fennel seeds and set aside.
3. Warm the rest of the oil in another pan and fry up the cod for 10 minutes, flipping halfway through until done.
4. Toss tomato sauce over heat to warm, then mix together the parsley, and serve atop the cod with a lemon slice.

# Baked Feta with Olive Tapenade

## Ingredients

- Baked pita or crusty bread to serve
- Feta cheese (6 oz.)
- Garlic (2 cloves)
- Green olives (0.33 c., sliced)
- Harissa paste (3 Tbsp.)
- Olive oil (3 Tbsp.)
- Parsley (3 Tbsp., fresh chopped)
- Roasted red peppers (16-oz. jar, drained)
- Salt (0.75 tsp.)
- Tomato paste (2 Tbsp.)
- Walnuts (0.5 c., halved)

## Instructions

1. In a blender, combine your peppers, 0.25 c. walnuts, harissa and tomato paste, garlic, and 0.5 tsp of your salt until mostly consistent. It doesn't have to be perfect, but should be well combined.
2. Take half of mixture into baking dish that has been sprayed with cooking spray. Top with half of your feta, then spoon the rest of the red pepper sauce atop it.
3. Top with the last of the feta and bake until bubbly, roughly 25 minutes. Broil for the last 2.
4. While that bakes, make your tapenade. This requires you to combine your remaining ingredients together.

5.  Remove mixture from oven and top with tapenade. Serve immediately with crusty bread or pita chips.

# Chapter 5: 30-Minutes or Less Meals

## Vegetarian Toss Together Mediterranean Pasta Salad

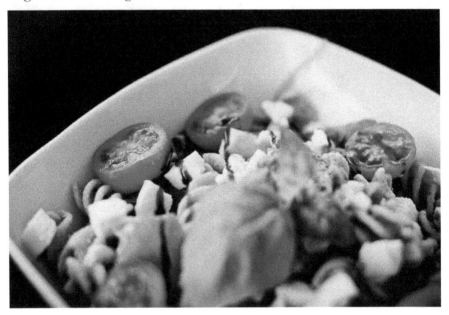

Ingredients

- Artichoke hearts (12 oz. jar, drained)
- Balsamic vinegar (2 Tbsp.)
- Kalamata olives (12-ounce jar, drained and chopped)
- Olive oil (2 Tbsp.)
- Pasta (8 oz., wheat)
- Salt to personal preference
- Sun-dried tomatoes in oil (1.5 oz. jar, drained)

Instructions

1. Prepare pasta according to packaging.

2. Mix together olives, tomatoes, and artichoke.

3. Drain pasta and add them to a bowl with artichoke mixture. Then, top with vinegar and olive oil, mix well, and serve warm.

## Vegetarian Aglio e Olio and Broccoli

Ingredients

- Olive oil (3 Tbsp.)
- Cayenne peppers (3)
- Garlic (3 cloves, sliced)
- Broccoli (1 head, prepared in florets)
- Spaghetti (7 oz. whole wheat)
- Salt to taste

Instructions

1. Boil water and prepare spaghetti according to instructions until al dente. Drain and reserve.

2. In a pan, heat up 1 Tbsp. of your olive oil at a moderate temperature, then toss in the garlic and peppers, sautéing until fragrant. Remove garlic from heat and set aside.

3. Toss broccoli into pan and cook for 4 minutes. Then toss in spaghetti, garlic, and remaining oil. Cook for an additional minute or two, then serve.

Cilantro and Garlic Baked Salmon

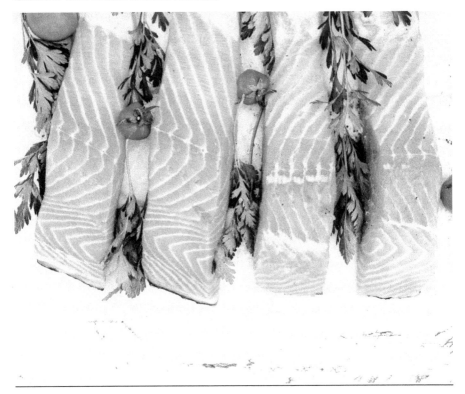

Ingredients

- Cilantro (stems trimmed)
- Garlic (4 cloves, chopped)
- Lime (0.5, cut into rounds)
- Lime juice (1 lime's worth)
- Olive oil (0.5 c.)
- Salmon fillet (2 pounds, skin removed)
- Salt to taste
- Tomato (cut into rounds)

Instructions

1. Allow salmon to come to room temp for 20 minutes while oven preheats to a temperature of 425 F.
2. While you wait, take a processor and combine garlic, cilantro, lime juice, and olive oil with a pinch of salt. Combine well.
3. Place fillet into baking pan that has been greased. Top with a light sprinkle of salt and pepper. Then spread cilantro sauce atop fillet, coating whole salmon. Top with tomato and lime.
4. Bake for 6 minutes per 0.5 inch of thickness (1-inch fillets take around 8-10 minutes). Let rest for 5-10 minutes out of the oven. Serve.

## Harissa Pasta

Ingredients

- Pasta (2 cups)
- Red bell pepper (1)
- Red onion (1)
- Pine nuts (2 Tbsp.)
- Harissa paste (2 Tbsp.)

Instructions

1. Roast onions and peppers with olive oil at 400F for 20 minutes. Remove from oven and dice.
2. Prepare pasta to instructions on package. While pasta cooks, toast your pine nuts until browned in frying pan.
3. Drain pasta, leaving a touch of the water. Then, add in diced roasted veggies and harissa. Serve topped with pine nuts.

# Chapter 6: 1-Hour-or-Less Meals

1 Hour Baked Cod

Ingredients

- Basil (0.5 tsp., dried)
- Bay leaf (1)
- Capers (1 small jar)
- Cod fillets (2 pounds)
- Fennel seeds (1 tsp., crushed)
- Garlic (1 clove, minced)
- Lemon juice (0.25 c., fresh)
- Olive oil (2 tsp)
- Onion (1, sliced)
- Orange juice (o.25 c., fresh)
- Orange peel (1 Tbsp.)
- Oregano (0.5 tsp., dried)
- Salt and pepper to personal preference
- White wine (1 c., dry)
- Whole tomatoes (16-oz. can, chopped and reserving juice)

Instructions

1. Warm oven to 375F.
2. In cast iron skillet, warm oil. Then, sauté your onion for 5 minutes. At this point, mix in all other ingredients but fish. Allow to simmer for 30 minutes.
3. Place fillets into skillet and top with most of the sauce. Allow to bake for 15 minutes until fish flakes.

Grilled Chicken Mediterranean Salad

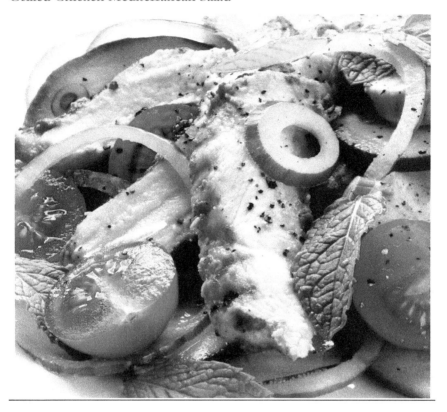

Ingredients

- Artichoke hearts (0.33 c., chopped)

- Balsamic vinegar (2 Tbsp.)

- Basil (1 tsp, dried)

- Chicken breasts (3, cut into bite-sized chunks)

- Cucumber (0.75 c., diced)

- Feta cheese (0.25 c.)

- Garlic (1 clove, minced)

- Greek yogurt (2 Tbsp.)

- Green onions (0.25 c., chopped)

- Kalamata olives (3 Tbsp., sliced)
- Kosher salt (0.5 tsp)
- Lemon juice (3 Tbsp + 1 tsp.)
- Olive oil (3 Tbsp. + 2 Tbsp.)
- Onion powder (0.5 tsp)
- Parsley (0.5 tsp)
- Pesto (4 tsp)
- Pinch of red pepper
- Roasted red pepper (6 Tbsp., sliced)
- Romaine (4 c., chopped)
- Shiitake mushrooms
- Spinach (4 c., chopped)
- Tomato (0.75 c., diced)
- White wine vinegar (4 tsp)

Instructions

1. Create your salad. Each plate should have a bed of romaine and spinach, topped with cucumber, tomato, artichoke, peppers, olives, and cheese.
2. Combine your tsp of lemon juice, wine vinegar, and pesto in a jar and shake to combine. Then, add in yogurt and 2 Tbsp. oil, mixing well until well-incorporated.
3. Prepare your chicken. Let it marinade in a mixture of 3 Tbsp. lemon juice, balsamic vinegar, remaining oil, and all seasonings for at least 30 minutes. Soak some wooden skewers in water during this time.
4. Make kebabs out of chicken and mushroom, alternating bite of chicken and bite of mushroom until chicken is gone. Grill for 10 to 15 minutes until done.
5. Drizzle salad with the vinaigrette, then place a kebab atop each. Serve.

# Lemon Herb Chicken and Potatoes One Pot Meal

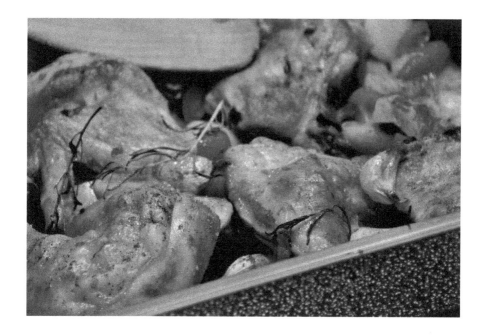

Ingredients

- Baby potatoes (8, halved)
- Basil (3 tsp, dried)
- Bell pepper (1, seeds removed and wedged)
- Chicken thighs (4, skin and bone on)
- Garlic (4 large cloves, crushed)
- Kalamata olives (4 Tbsp., pitted)
- Lemon juice (1 lemon's worth)
- Olive oil (3 Tbsp.)
- Oregano (2 tsp, dried)

- Parsley (2 tsp, dried)
- Red onion (wedged)
- Red wine vinegar (1 Tbsp.)
- Salt (2 tsp)
- Zucchini (1 large, sliced)
- Lemons for garnish

Instructions

1. Combine juice from lemon, 2 Tbsp. olive oil, vinegar, seasonings, and garlic into dish. Pour half to reserve for later, then place chicken in half. Let sit for 15 minutes (or overnight if you would like to prep the day before)
2. Warm oven to 430F. Sear chicken in cast iron skillet in remaining olive oil, about 4 minutes per side. Drain all but 1 Tbsp. of fat.
3. Place all veggies around the thighs. Top with remaining marinade and combine well to cover everything.
4. Cover pan and bake for 35 minutes until soft and chicken is to temperature. Then, broil for 5 minutes or until golden brown. Top with olives and lemon to serve.

## Vegetarian Mediterranean Quiche

Ingredients

- Butter (2 Tbsp.)
- Cheddar cheese (1 c., shredded)
- Eggs (4 large)
- Feta (0.33 c.)
- Garlic (2 cloves, minced)
- Kalamata olives (0.25 c., sliced)
- Milk (1.25 c.)
- Onion (1, diced)
- Oregano (1 tsp, dried)
- Parsley (1 tsp, dried)
- Pie crust (1, prepared)
- Red pepper (1, diced)
- Salt and pepper to personal preference
- Spinach (2 c., fresh)
- Sun dried tomatoes (0.5 c.)

Instructions

1. Soak sun-dried tomatoes in boiling water for 5 minutes before draining and chopping.
2. Prepare a pie dish with a crust, fluting the edges.
3. In a skillet, melt your butter, then cook your garlic and onions in it until they become fragrant. Combine in the red peppers for another 3 minutes until softened. Then, toss in your spinach, olives, and seasoning. Cook until the spinach wilts, about 5 minutes. Take it off of the heat and toss

in your feta and tomatoes. Then, carefully place mixture into the crust, spreading it into a nice, even layer.

4.  Mix milk, eggs, and half of cheddar cheese together. Pour it into the crust. Then, top with cheddar.

5.  Bake for 50 minutes at 375 f. until crust is browned and egg is done.

Herbed Lamb and Veggies

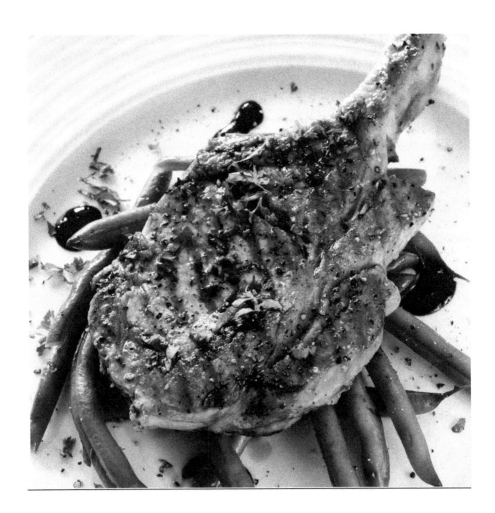

Ingredients

- Bell pepper (2, any color, seeds removed and cut into bite-sized chunks)
- Lamb cutlets (8 lean)
- Mint (2 Tbsp., fresh, chopped)
- Olive oil (1 Tbsp.)
- Red onion (1, wedged)
- Sweet potato (1 large, peeled, and chunked)
- Thyme (1 Tbsp., fresh, chopped)
- Zucchini (2, chunked)

Instructions

1. Assemble your veggies onto a baking sheet and coat with oil and black pepper. Bake at 400F for 25 minutes.
2. As veggies bake, trim fat from the lamb. Then, combine the herbs with a bit of freshly ground pepper. Coat the lamb in the seasoning.
3. Remove veggies, flip, and push to one side of pan. Then, arrange your cutlets onto the baking pan as well. Bake for 10 minutes, flip, then cook an additional 10 minutes. Combine well, then serve.

Chicken and Couscous Mediterranean Wraps

Ingredients

- Parsley (1 c., fresh and chopped)
- Olive oil (3 Tbsp.)

- Garlic (2 tsp, minced)
- Salt (pinch)
- Pepper (pinch)
- Chicken tenders (1 pound)
- Tomato (1, chopped)
- Cucumber (1, chopped)
- Spinach wraps (4 1o-inch)
- Water (0.5 c)
- Mint (0.5 c., fresh chopped)
- Lemon juice (0.25 c.)
- Couscous (0.33 c.)

Instructions

1. Cook couscous in boiling water according to directions on package.
2. Mix together your lemon juice, oil, garlic, salt and pepper, mint, and parsley.
3. Coat chicken in 1 Tbsp. of your mixture from previous step and top with a pinch of salt. Cook in skillet until completely cooked, usually just a few minutes per side.
4. Wait for chicken to cool, then chop into bites.
5. Pour the remainder of your parsley mixture into the couscous with cucumbers and tomato bits.
6. Place 0.75 c. of couscous mixture into a tortilla, then spread chicken atop it, rolling them up and serving.

# Sheet Pan Shrimp

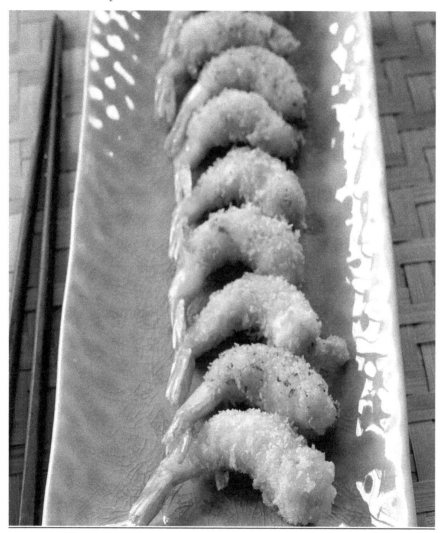

Ingredients

*For shrimp*

- Feta cheese (0.5 c.)

- Fingerling potatoes (2 c., halved)

- Green beans (6 oz., trimmed)

- Olive oil (3 Tbsp.)

- Pepper (1 tsp)

- Red onion (1 medium, sliced)

- Red pepper (1 medium, sliced)

- Salt (1 tsp)

- Shrimp (1 lb., deveined and peeled)

*For Marinade*

- Garlic (1 Tbsp., minced) Oregano (0.5 tsp)

- Greek yogurt (1 c.)

- Lemon juice (2 Tbsp.)

- Paprika (0.5 tsp)

- Parsley (2 Tbsp., chopped)

Instructions

1. Combine all marinade ingredients and set aside.
2. Take shrimp in a bowl with 0.5 c. of the marinade. Let them sit for 30 minutes.
3. During rest time, set up your baking sheet with foil or parchment, and prepare your veggies. Chop them up and toss onto baking sheet, drizzling them with the olive oil and giving them a quick sprinkle of salt and pepper. Bake for roughly 20 minutes at 400F, then remove from oven. Take out all green beans and set to the side.
4. Place shrimp in one layer across the pan and bake for an additional 10 minutes until shrimp is done. Serve with veggies and shrimp in bowls, topped with 2 Tbsp. feta and a spoonful of yogurt marinade.

## Mediterranean Mahi Mahi

Ingredients

- Basil (6 leaves, freshly chopped)
- Capers (4 Tbsp.)
- Garlic (2 cloves, chopped)
- Italian seasoning (pinch)
- Kalamata olives (25, chopped)
- Lemon juice (1 tsp)
- Mahi mahi (1 pound)
- Olive oil (2 Tbsp.)
- Onion (0.5, chopped)
- Parmesan cheese (3 Tbsp.)
- Diced tomatoes (15 oz. can)
- White wine (0.25 c.)

Instructions

1. Warm olive oil in a pan and then cook onions until translucent. Toss in garlic and seasoning and stir to mix well. Then, add in your can of tomatoes, wine, olives, lemon, and roughly half of the chopped basil. Drop heat down and toss in parmesan cheese. Cook until bubbling.
2. Put fish into a baking pan, then top with the sauce. Bake for 20 minutes at 425 F until fish is to temperature.

# Chapter 7: Slow Cooker Meals

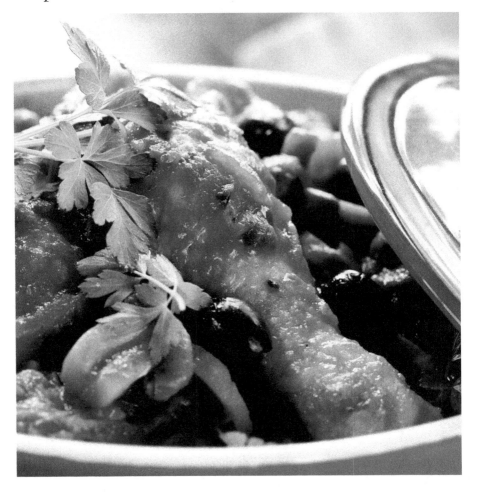

Slow Cooker Mediterranean Chicken

Ingredients

- Bay leaf (1)
- Capers (1 Tbsp.)
- Chicken broth (0.5 c.)

- Chicken thighs (2 pounds, bone and skin removed)
- Garlic (3 cloves, minced)
- Kalamata olives (1 c.)
- Olive oil (1 Tbsp.)
- Oregano (1 tsp)
- Roasted red pepper (1 c.)
- Rosemary (1 tsp, dried)
- Salt and pepper to taste
- Sweet onion (1, thinly sliced)
- Thyme (1 tsp, dried)
- Optional fresh lemon wedges to juice for serving

Instructions

1. Sauté the chicken in olive oil to brown on both sides, then remove it from the pan. Then, sauté the onions and garlic as well until beginning to soften, roughly 5 minutes.
2. Put chicken, onion, garlic, and all other ingredients into a slow cooker and leave it to cook for 4 hours on low. Season to taste.

# Slow Cooker Vegetarian Mediterranean Stew

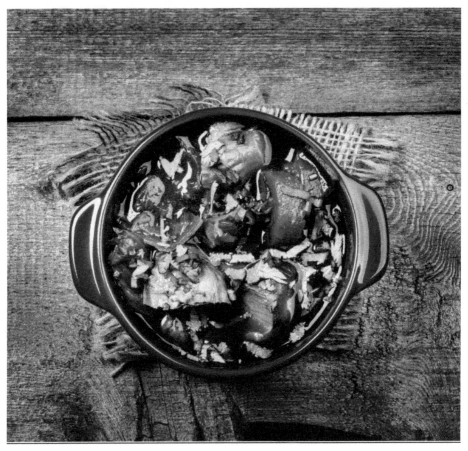

Ingredients

- Carrot (0.75 c., chopped)

- Chickpeas (15 oz. can)

- Crushed red pepper (0.5 tsp)

- Fire-roasted diced tomatoes (2 14-oz. cans)

- Garlic (4 cloves, minced)

- Ground pepper (0.25 tsp)

- Kale (8 c., chopped)

- Lemon juice (1 Tbsp.)
- Olive oil ( 3 Tbsp.)
- Onion (1, chopped)
- Oregano (1 tsp)
- Salt (0.75 tsp)
- Vegetable broth (3 c.)
- Basil leaves (garnish)
- Lemon wedges (garnish)

Instructions

1. Mix tomatoes, onion, carrot, broth, seasonings, and garlic into the slow cooker. Cook on low for 6 hours.
2. Take out 0.25 c. of the liquid in the slow cooker after 6 hours and transfer it to a bowl. Take out 2 Tbsp. of chickpeas and mash them with the liquid until nice and smooth.
3. Combine mash, kale, juice from lemon, and whole chickpeas. Cook for about 30 minutes, until kale is tender, then serve garnished with the basil leaves and lemon wedges.

# Vegetarian Slow Cooker Quinoa

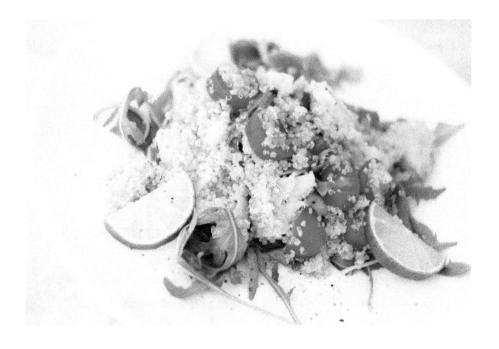

Ingredients

- Arugula (4 c.)

- Chickpeas (1 15.5 oz. can, rinsed and drained)

- Feta cheese (0.5 c)

- Garlic (2 cloves, minced)

- Kalamata olives (12, halved)

- Kosher salt (0.75 tsp)

- Lemon juice (2 tsp)

- Olive oil (2.25 Tbsp.)

- Oregano (2 Tbsp., fresh and coarsely chopped

- Quinoa (1.5 c., uncooked)
- Red onion (1 c., sliced)
- Roasted red pepper (0.5 c., drained and chopped)
- Vegetable stock (2.25 c.)

Instructions

1. Mix your broth with the onion, garlic, quinoa, chickpeas, and 1.5 tsp of olive oil. Sprinkle half of the salt atop it. Mix and cook on low until quinoa is done, roughly 3 or 4 hours.
2. Turn off the slow cooker and mix well. In a separate bowl, combine remaining olive oil, salt, and lemon juice together. Then, mix that into the slow cooker, along with the peppers.
3. Combine in the arugula and leave until the greens start to wilt. Serve, topping with feta, oregano, and olives.

## Slow-Cooked Chicken and Chickpea Soup

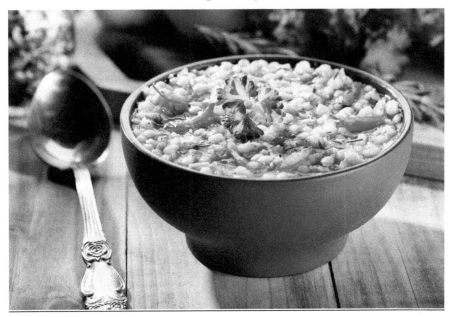

Ingredients

- Artichoke hearts (14 oz. can, drained and chopped)
- Bay leaf (1)
- Cayenne (0.25 tsp)
- Chicken thighs (2 lbs., skins removed)
- Cumin (4 tsp)
- Diced tomatoes (1 15-ounce can)
- Dried chickpeas (1.5 c., allow to soak overnight)
- Garlic cloves (4, chopped)
- Olives (o.25 c., halved)
- Paprika (4 tsp)
- Pepper (0.25 tsp)
- Salt (0.5 tsp)

- Tomato paste (2 Tbsp.)
- Water (4 c.)
- Yellow onion (chopped)
- Parsley or cilantro (garnish)

Instructions

1. Drain your soaked chickpeas and place them into your slow cooker (large preferred). Mix in the water, onions and garlic, tomatoes (undrained), tomato paste, and all seasonings. Combine well, then add in the chicken.
2. Leave it to cook for 8 hours at low, or 4 at high.
3. Remove the chicken and allow it to cool on a cutting board. At the same time, remove the bay leaf, then add in the artichoke and olives. Season with additional salt if necessary to taste. Chop up chicken, removing the bones, and then mix it back into the soup. Serve the soup with the parsley or cilantro garnishing the top.

Slow Cooked Brisket

Ingredients

- Beef broth (0.5 c.)
- Brisket (3 lbs.)
- Cold water (0.25 c.)
- Fennel bulbs (2, cored, trimmed, and cut into wedges)
- Flour
- Italian seasoning (3 tsp)
- Italian seasoning diced tomatoes (14.5 oz. can)
- Lemon peel (1 tsp., fine shreds)
- Olives (0.5 c.)
- Parsley for garnish
- Pepper (pinch)
- Salt (pinch)

Instructions

1. Trim meat, then season with 1 tsp Italian seasoning. Put it in slow cooker with the cut-up fennel on top.
2. Mix together the tomatoes, broth, peel, olives, salt and pepper, and the last of the Italian seasoning.
3. Cook at low for 10 hours, or high for 5.
4. Take meat out of the cooker and reserve all juice. Arrange meat with veggies on a serving platter.
5. Remove fat from top of the juices.
6. Take 2 c. of juices in saucepan. Mix together water and flour, then combine it into the juice. Cook until gravy forms.
7. Serve meat topped with gravy and garnish with parsley.

# Vegan Bean Soup with Spinach

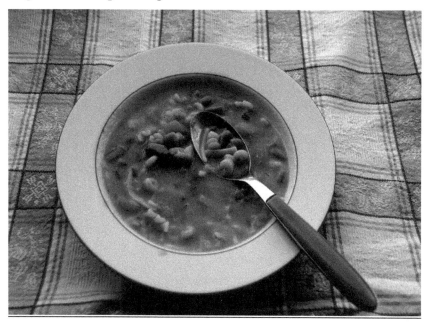

Ingredients

- Vegetable broth (3 14-oz. cans)
- Tomato puree (15 oz. can)
- Great Northern or White beans (15 oz. can)
- White rice (0.5 c)
- Onion (0.5 c., chopped)
- Garlic (2 cloves, minced)
- Basil (1 tsp., dried)
- Pinch of salt
- Pinch of pepper
- Kale or spinach (8 c., chopped)

Instructions

1. Mix everything but leafy greens together in your slow cooker. Cook for 5 or 7 hours on low, or 2.5 hours on high.
2. Toss in leafy greens. Wait for them to wilt and serve.

# Moroccan Lentil Soup

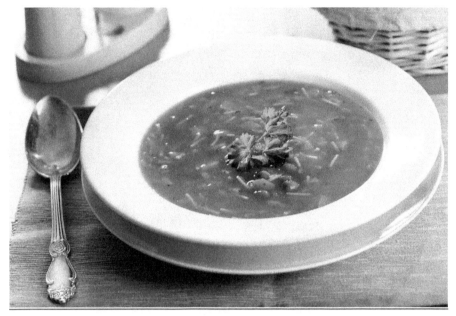

## Ingredients

- Carrots (2 c., chopped)
- Cauliflower (3 c.)
- Cinnamon (0.25 tsp)
- Cumin (1 tsp)
- Diced tomato (28 oz.)
- Fresh cilantro (0.5 c.)
- Fresh spinach (4 c.)
- Garlic (4 cloves, minced)
- Ground coriander (1 tsp)
- Lemon juice (2 Tbsp.)
- Lentils (1.75 c.)
- Olive oil (2 tsp)

- Onion (2 c., chopped)
- Pepper (pinch)
- Tomato paste (2 Tbsp.)
- Turmeric (1 tsp)
- Vegetable broth (6 c.)
- Water (2 c.)

Instructions

1. Mix everything but spinach, cilantro, and lemon juice. Cook until lentils soften. This will be 4-5 hours if you use high heat, or 10 hours on low.
2. Mix spinach when just 30 minutes remains on cook time.
3. Just before serving, top with cilantro and lemon juice.

# Chapter 8: Vegetarian and Vegan Meals

## Vegetarian Greek Stuffed Mushrooms

Ingredients

- Cherry tomatoes (0.5 c., quartered)
- Feta cheese (0.33 c.)
- Garlic (1 clove, mixed)
- Ground pepper (0.5 tsp)
- Kalamata olives (2 Tbsp.)
- Olive oil (3 Tbsp.)
- Oregano (1 Tbsp., fresh and roughly chopped)
- Portobello mushrooms (4, cleaned with stems and gills taken out)
- Salt (0.25 tsp)
- Spinach (1 c., chopped)

Instructions

1. Begin by setting your oven. This recipe requires 400F for baking.
2. Mix together your salt and 0.25 tsp pepper, garlic, and 2 Tbsp. of oil, and use it to cover your mushrooms, inside and out.
3. Set the mushrooms onto your baking pan and allow it to cook for 10 minutes.
4. Mix together your remaining ingredients and combine well. Then, when the mushrooms are done, remove them from the oven and then fill them up with your filling.
5. Allow to cook for another 10 minutes.

# Vegetarian Cheesy Artichoke and Spinach Stuffed Squash

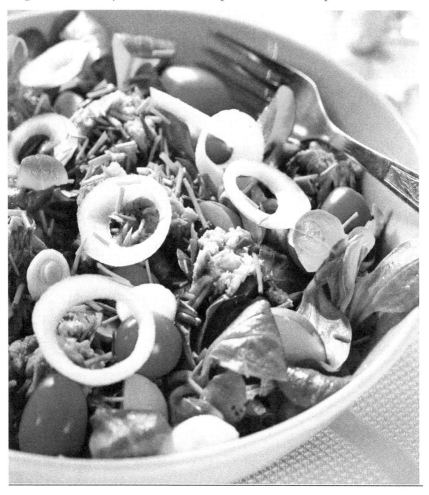

Ingredients

- Artichoke Hearts (10 oz., frozen—thawed and chopped up)
- Baby spinach (5 oz.)
- Cream cheese (4 oz., softened)
- Parmesan cheese (0.5 c.)
- Pepper (pinch to taste)
- Red pepper and basil (for garnish)

- Salt (pinch to taste)
- Spaghetti squash (1, cut in half and cleaned out of seeds)
- Water (3 Tbsp.)

Instructions

1. Microwave your squash, flat side down, with 2 Tbsp. of your water uncovered for 10-15 minutes.
2. Mix together your spinach and water into a skillet until they begin to wilt. Then drain and reserve for later.
3. Preheat your oven set to broil with the rack at the upper 1/3 point.
4. Remove flesh from squash with a fork, then place the shells onto a sheet for the oven. Then stir in your artichoke, cheeses, and a pinch of salt and pepper to the squash flesh. Combine thoroughly, then split it between the two shells. Broil for 3 minutes and top with red pepper and basil to taste.

# Vegan Mediterranean Buddha Bowl

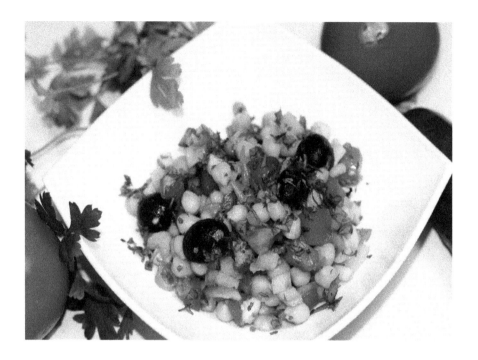

Ingredients

*For the chickpeas*

- Chickpeas (1 can, rinsed, drained, and skinned)
- Olive oil (1 tsp)
- Pinch of salt and pepper
- Dried basil (0.25 tsp)
- Garlic powder (0.25 tsp)

*For the quinoa*

- Quinoa (0.5 c.)
- Water (1 c.)

*For the salad*

- Bell pepper (1, color of choice, seeded, stemmed, and chopped to bite-sized bits)
- Cucumbers (2, peeled and chopped)
- Grape tomatoes (1 c., halved)
- Hummus (0.5 c.)
- Kalamata olives (0.5 c.)
- Lettuce (2 c. – can sub in field greens, spinach, kale, or any other leafy greens)

Instructions

1. Set your oven up to prepare for baking. It should be at 0400F. Then, mix the ingredients for the chickpeas together, coating them evenly with the seasoning.
2. Put chickpeas in single layer and put them onto the baking sheet. Roast for 30 minutes with an occasional mixing and rotation of the pan to allow them all to cook evenly. Allow them to cool.
3. Start preparing the quinoa and water in a microwave-safe bowl. Combine the water and quinoa and microwave, covered, for 4 minutes. Then stir and microwave for 2 minutes longer. Give it one final stir and leave it to rest in the microwave for another minute or two.
4. Begin assembling your salad. Begin with the greens at the bottom, then top with tomatoes, cucumbers, bell pepper, olives, chickpeas, and then quinoa. Finally, top with a dollop of hummus to serve.

## Vegan Mediterranean Pasta

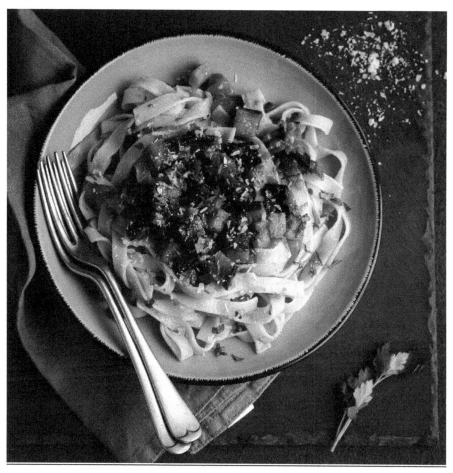

Ingredients

- Artichokes (0.5 c.)
- Basil leaves (0.25 c., torn)
- Garlic cloves (2-3 to taste, minced)
- Grape tomatoes (2 c., halved)
- Kalamata olives (10, pitted)
- Olive oil (1 Tbsp.)

- Pasta (8 oz.)
- Red pepper (0.25 tsp.)
- Salt and pepper to taste
- Spinach (4 c.)
- Tomato paste (4 Tbsp.)
- Vegetable broth (1 c.)

Instructions

1. Prepare your pasta based on the instructions provided. Keep 1 c. of the water for later use and then set the pasta aside.
2. While preparing your pasta, take the time to warm a large skillet with oil. Then, sauté your garlic and red pepper for 30 seconds or so. Combine in the tomato paste and cook for another minute. At that point, mix in your tomatoes, your seasoning, your artichokes and olives, and your broth. Let it cook until tomatoes start to break down.
3. Mix in the pasta to the tomato mixture. Let it cook another 2 minutes and add reserved pasta water if too dry.
4. Add in spinach and basil and cook until wilted.
5. Remove from heat and serve.

## Vegetarian Zucchini Lasagna Rolls

Ingredients

- Basil (2 Tbsp., fresh)
- Egg (1, lightly beaten)
- Frozen spinach (10-ounce package, thawed and dried)
- Garlic (1 clove)
- Marinara sauce (0.75 c.)
- Olive oil (2 tsp)
- Parmesan cheese (3 Tbsp.)
- Pinch each of salt and pepper
- Ricotta (1.33 c.)
- Shredded mozzarella cheese (8 Tbsp.)
- Zucchini (2, trimmed)

Instructions

1. Prepare two baking sheets with cooking spray. Then set the oven to 425F.
2. Cut up your zucchini into strips lengthwise into 1/8 inch thick pieces. A mandolin will make this easier.
3. Prepare zucchini coated in oil with salt and pepper, then set up a flat layer across the bottom of the prepared pan.
4. Bake zucchini for 10 minutes until it begins to soften.
5. Mix together 2 Tbsp. mozzarella and 1 Tbsp. of parmesan. Then, in another bowl, combine egg, ricotta, spinach, garlic, and the remainder of the cheese. Toss in a pinch of salt and pepper and mix well.
6. Set up an 8-inch square casserole dish with 0.25 c. marinara spread across the bottom.
7. Take your zucchini that has been softened and begin to roll it. To do this, you will need to put 1 Tbsp. of ricotta mix at the bottom of your strip, then roll. Put the seam down in the marinara-covered bottom. Do this for all pieces of zucchini.
8. Cover the rolls with the remainder of your marinara sauce and top with the cheese mix.
9. Bake until bubbling, roughly 20 minutes. Rest for 5 minutes and top with basil.

# Vegetarian Breakfast Sandwich

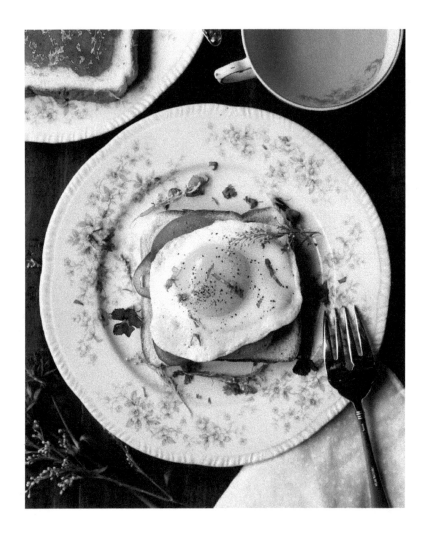

Ingredients

- Sandwich thins (2)
- Olive oil (2 Tbsp. + 1 tsp)
- Rosemary (1 Tbsp. fresh, or 0.5 tsp dried)
- Eggs (2)

- Spinach leaves (1 c.)
- Tomato (0.5, sliced thinly)
- Feta (2 Tbsp.)
- Pinch of salt and pepper

Instructions

1. Warm oven to 375F. Separate your sandwich thins and coat with olive oil. Bake for 5 minutes until beginning to crisp up.
2. Warm skillet with last tsp of olive oil. Break eggs into pan and cook until whites are set. Then, break the yolks and flip to finish cooking.
3. Put bottoms of the bread onto serving plates. Then, top with spinach, the tomato, one egg each, followed by the feta. Sprinkle with salt and pepper, then top with remaining bread.

Vegan Breakfast Toast

Ingredients

- Bread of choice (verify that it is vegan—2 slices)
- Spice blend of choice
- Arugula (handful)
- Tomato (1, cut into rounds)
- Chopped olives (1 Tbsp.)
- Cucumber (0.5, cut into rounds)
- Hummus (0.25 c.)

Instructions

1. Toast up your bread. Then spread the hummus across, season it, and top with all toppings split between the pieces.

# Vegetarian Shakshouka

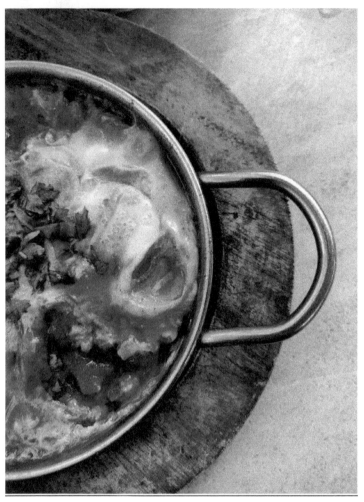

## Ingredients

- Chopped parsley (1 Tbsp.)
- Diced Tomatoes (15 oz. can)
- Eggs (4)
- Garlic (2 cloves)

- Olive oil (2 Tbsp.)
- Onion (1—sliced)
- Red bell peppers (2, sliced thinly)
- Salt and pepper to taste
- Spicy harissa (1 tsp)
- Sugar (1 tsp)

Instructions

1. Warm oil in a cast iron pan. Sauté your peppers and onions until they have begun to soften, giving them a stir every now and then to prevent sticking. Add in the garlic for another minute.
2. Put in tomatoes, sugar, and harissa, leaving it to simmer for the next 7 minutes.
3. Season it to taste. Then, add in small indentations into the mixture in the pan, cracking an egg in each indentation that you make. Cover up the pot and allow it to cook until egg whites are done.
4. **Cover with parsley and serve with bread.**

# PART II

# Chapter 1: The Fundamentals of a Low Sugar Diet for Diabetics

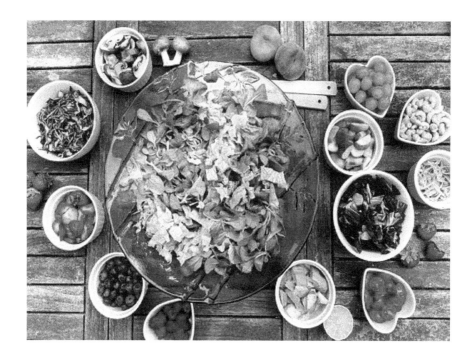

For people with diabetes, eating can be quite a challenge. After all, it's not easy dealing with the various recommendations made by doctors. The fact is that the following recommended guidelines are essential to keeping your diabetes in check.

You see, it's important to ensure that your blood sugar levels remain in check. One of the easiest and most effective ways to do this is by keeping your sugar and carb intake as low as possible. So, let's take a look at how this occurs when you go on the low-sugar and low-carb, diabetic diet.

Firstly, when you consume carbs and sugars, these are converted into glucose in the bloodstream as the liver metabolizes them. Since carbs are used as a source of energy, the body needs to secrete insulin from the pancreas in order to break down glucose and send it into the cells as functional energy. Then, the body mixes oxygen to create ATP. This is the source of energy that helps you power your body's entire system.

All is good until there is an excess of glucose in the body. When this occurs, the body stores excess glucose as fat. However, there comes a point where the body just can't keep up. This is where insulin resistance happens. In a nutshell, your cells simply stop accepting any more glucose as there is simply too much glucose in the bloodstream.

These are the spikes in blood sugar levels.

This is where the low-carb, low-sugar diet makes a huge difference in your overall health management plan. The rationale is that when you restrict the number of carbs and sugar that you consume, you are basically giving your body the chance to process what's already in the bloodstream and in storage. So, you are creating a deficit that forces the body to use up what it's already stored.

This is how you can get your blood sugar levels in check.

In a manner of speaking, what you are doing is giving your body a break. Therefore, the body has a chance to catch up. When your body eventually catches up, you end up reducing your overall blood sugar levels. In addition, medication is much more effective as there are fewer carbs and glucose to process.

At first, it can be a bit of a psychological shock to think that you have to go on a low-carb, low-sugar diet. In fact, most people think they have to live on lettuce for the rest of their lives. What you will find is that this diet embraces a large number of foods that are very low in carbs and sugar. As a result, you can eat healthy and tasty at the same time.

However, the secret is knowing which foods promote low blood sugar levels. When you discover these foods, you'll find that keeping your diabetes in check doesn't have to be tough. You can still enjoy delicious foods with zero guilt.

Now that's a plan!

# Chapter 2: Benefits of a Low Sugar Diet for Diabetics

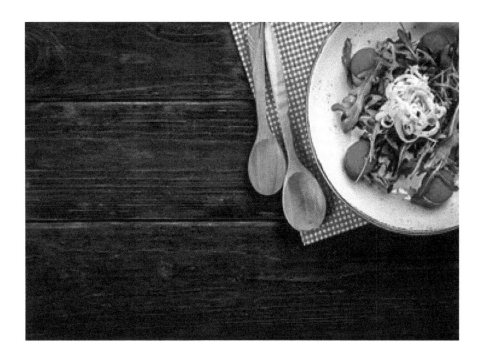

The low-sugar, low-carb diet is filled with a number of benefits that diabetics can obtain. The best part is that you don't need to wait for an extended period of time to see the benefits. In fact, you can see benefits within a few days of trying out the diet. This is what makes the diet itself so encouraging.

So, here is a list of five benefits you can expect when going on the low-sugar diet.

### 1. Reduction in blood sugar levels

Naturally, this is the most immediate benefit of this diet. As mentioned earlier, when you reduce the amount of carbs and sugar, your body will begin to use up what's already stored in the system. This is why you can begin to see a reduction in your blood sugar levels within a few days. Over time, your blood sugar levels will begin to normalize. So, the diet, along with medication, will prove to be quite effective.

## 2. Weight loss

Another benefit is weight loss. Since the body converts glucose into fat when it's stored, a reduction in your carb and sugar consumption will force your body to convert stored fat into energy. This is why folks who go on the low-carb diet begin to see weight loss after a few weeks. While this result isn't immediate, it is almost certain that you'll see weight loss, especially if you are overweight.

## 3. Increased levels of energy

One of the symptoms that accompany diabetes is low levels of energy. This is due to the imbalance that occurs in the metabolism. Since the metabolism cannot keep up with the amount of carbs and sugar in the bloodstream, it does not produce energy as efficiently as it could. As a result, there are lower levels of energy. When you essentially force your body to process stored up fat, your metabolism becomes more efficient in producing energy. The end result is a boost in energy levels. So, don't be surprised if you find at you feel more energetic after a few days.

## 4. Hormonal regulation

Hormones tend to go out of whack when there are increased levels of blood sugar. For instance, insulin is the first hormone that goes haywire. However, other hormones are affected as well, such as cortisol (it is associated with weight gain) or epinephrine (used to breakdown and release nutrients in the blood). These hormones tend to work inefficiently when there is a high level of blood sugar. As a result, you may not be getting the most nutrition out of the foods you eat.

## 5.  Improved cognitive function

Sugar, in general, works like a fuel in your body. So, when you consume a large amount of sugar, you get the rush that can power you through a given time period. However, sugar is a very poor fuel as your brain burns right through it. The end result is a severe crash afterward. Over time, your brain builds up "gunk." This gunk limits the brain's capabilities. As such, when you replace sugar with other types of fuels, such as vegetable-based carbs, then your brain produces energy more effectively. It's like putting diesel into an unleaded engine. Sure, the car will run, but it will run poorly. This is why many folks on the low-sugar diet report improved cognitive abilities, thereby reducing the phenomenon known as "brain fog."

With these benefits, you can't go wrong with the low-sugar diet!

# Chapter 3: Savory Recipe Ideas

Savory Idea #1: Tangy Cabbage Treat
Number of people served: 4
Time you'll need: 33 to 37 minutes


Calories: 253

Fats: 22.8 g
Proteins: 7.9 g
Carbs: 4.7 g


**What you'll require:**

- Jalapeno Peppers (two, chopped)
- Cabbage (one Head)
- Pepper & salt (as preferred)
- Onion (one, chopped)
- Bacon (six, strips)


**What you need to do:**

1. Firstly, cook bacon as per the directions on the pack. While you allow the bacon to reach its optimal point, ready cabbage, and onions by chopping into smaller bite-sized morsels.
2. Once the bacon has been prepared to your preference, take it out of the pan and toss the onion and cabbage in. Please ensure to mix up everything with the leftover grease from the bacon while simmering in low fire.
3. Next, get the jalapenos ready by cutting up into pieces as small as you like. Feel free to throw in with the other elements.
4. After the vegetables have reached their optimal point, take the crispy bacon and crumble over the entire mix. Add pepper & salt, along with any other low-carb or low-sugar spices.
5. Lastly, toss everything around until the entire mix is thoroughly even. Serve and enjoy!

Savory Idea #2: Low-carb Egg &Veggie Bites

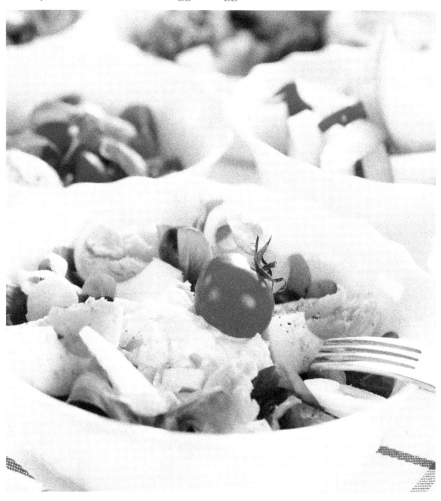

Number of people served: 6

Time you'll need: 11 to 14 minutes

Calories: 21.8

Fats: 3.7 g

Proteins: 4.3 g

Carbs: 1.8 g

**What you'll require:**

- Bell Pepper (75 g, Chopped)
- Cucumber (45 g, Chopped)
- Spinach (225 g, Chopped)
- Tomato (75 g, Chopped)
- Eggs (three)
- Salt (as preferred)

**What you need to do:**

1. To get started, set up oven to 180 degrees Celsius along with a muffin tray. The smaller trays are better as they allow for smaller portions if you wish.
2. Next, use a mixing container and place eggs (cracked) inside. Whisk briskly until they are thoroughly mixed.
3. Now, coat trays with your choice of grease (for instance, non-stick spray). Please ensure to leave some extra for the vegetables (chopped)
4. Then, place eggs in the spaces in the tray and toss in vegetables are per your preference. Please make sure to stir so that the mix is distributed evenly. Then, place in the heat for roughly 11 to 14 minutes.
5. Lastly, make sure to check the mixture is cooked all the way through. Serve as a breakfast treat or yummy snack.

Savory Idea #3: Yummy Chicken Dee-light

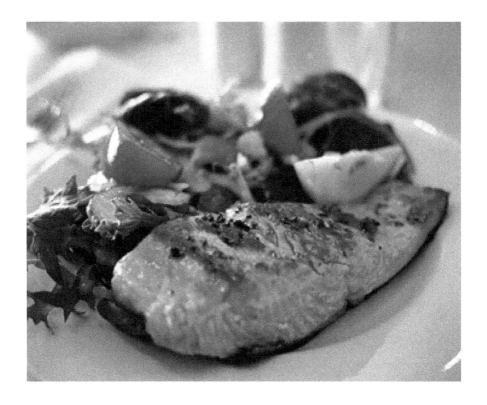

Number of people served: 2

Time you'll need: 35 to 40 minutes

Calories: 794.7

Fats: 39.1 g

Proteins: 44.2 g

Carbs: 3.3 g

**What you'll require:**

- Rosemary Leaves (10 g)
- Pepper & salt (as preferred)
- Garlic (cloves, six, minced)
- Chicken Breast (455 g boneless & skinless)
- Cheddar Cheese (70 g, shredded)
- Butter (55 g)

**What you need to do:**

1. Firstly, set up your oven to a temperature of approximately 190 degrees Celsius. While the oven gain temperature, prepare a tray with grease (your choice).
2. Next, add seasoning to chicken to your liking.
3. Then, begin to prepare garlic butter. Take pan or skillet and set to medium fire on the range. Once the butter has thoroughly melted, toss in garlic and let cook for roughly five to six minutes. Once this time has passed, garlic should be brownish, but make sure it is not burnt. Now, cover chicken with this butter & garlic mix.
4. Once this mix is prepared, set into the oven for about ½ an hour. Make sure to check the chicken so that it is fully cooked all the way through to the center. Once this has been achieved, add cheese as a topping. Allow to melt.
5. Serve by adding some more butter & garlic mix on top. Enjoy!

Savory Idea #4: Low-carb Fried Chicken Surprise

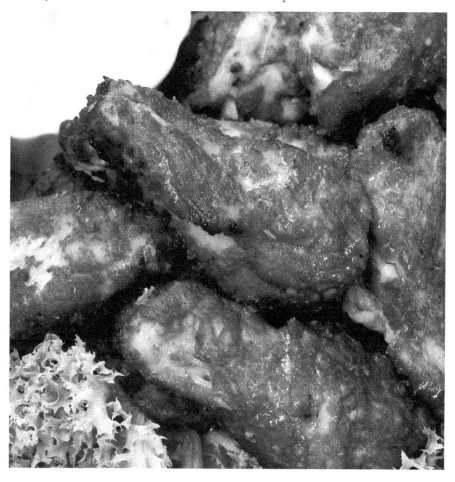

Number of people served: 6

Time you'll need: 33 minutes

Calories: 768

Fats: 54.1 g

Proteins: 59.2 g

Carbs: 1.9 g

**What you'll require:**

- Pork (rinds, 85 g)
- Pepper & salt (as preferred)
- Lard (according to need)
- Egg (one)
- Chicken (thighs, six)

**What you need to do:**

1. First, heat up iron pan or skillet on a range top. Then, place eggs in a mixing container for whisking.
2. Next, prepare rinds by crumbling. Upon completion, coat chicken pieces with egg (you can use a brush or dip) and season as per your liking with salt & pepper.
3. Now, take covered chicken pieces and roll over in the rind crumbs. Do this for every piece.
4. After, add in about half an inch of lard (or cooking oil) into pan or skillet. Wait until it reaches the boiling point. Then, place chicken pieces into the fire. Leave for about four to six minutes on each side. Please make sure they are cooked all the way through.
5. Please ensure to turn chicken around at least twice to ensure proper cooking. Serve with a side of crispy veggies or veggie chips.

Savory Idea #5: Low-Sugar Beef Explosion

Number of people served: 4

Time you'll need: one hour

Calories: 331

Fats: 26.7 g

Proteins: 18.7 g

Carbs: 2.1 g

**What you'll require:**

- Garlic (cloves, two, chopped)
- Coconut grounds (55 g)
- Onions (green, three)
- Coconut Oil (45 g)
- Ginger (10 g, grated)
- Steak (Flat-iron, 455 g)

**What you need to do:**

1. First, get steak ready by cutting it up into long, thin slices. Upon completion, place into a large freezer bag so that you can add ginger, coconut grounds, and garlic. Then, place into refrigeration so it can marinate for about one hour's time.
2. Next, put a pan or skillet to heat. Add oil for the meat. Heat up for about three to four minutes until it is at boiling point. Then, toss in steak and let sit until thoroughly cooked. This should take about five to seven minutes.
3. After, add in onions (green) to give the flavor a kick. Let everything sit for a minute or two until the texture is as per your liking.
4. Lastly, take some of the marinade from the freezer bag and add in right before turning off the fire. This will add an extra kick. Serve over zucchini pasta or low-carb couscous.

Savory Idea #6: Tangy Pork Extravaganza

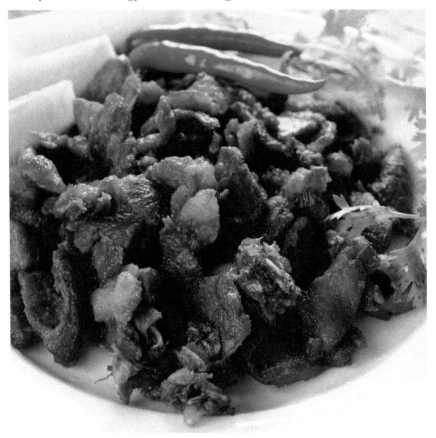

Number of people served: 4

Time you'll need: 34 to 37 minutes

Calories: 466.1

Fats: 32.3 g

Proteins: 47.2 g

Carbs: 2.7 g

**What you'll require:**

- Stock (chicken, 55 g)

- Pepper (7.5 g)
- Pork (chops, four)
- Milk (202 g)
- Coriander (9 g)
- Thyme (dried, 14.5 g)
- Garlic (cloves, two, minced)
- Butter (47 g)
- Salt (14.5 g)
- Oregano (dried, 14.5 g)

**What you need to do:**

1. First, get chops ready by placing them on a baking sheet. Sprinkle with pepper & salt to season. Please ensure that seasoning is evenly distributed to guarantee flavor. Let sit for one hour. Once time has passed, carefully rinse chops of excess fluid.

2. Next, set the pan to high heat on range top. Place garlic & butter to stir. Once the garlic is fully transparent, the time has come to add in chops on top.

3. Once chops are placed, cook them through for roughly four to six minutes on both sides. Then, let simmer for another minute, or so, to enable flavors to combine. Remove and set aside.

4. Then, on low fire, throw in stock (chicken), and some milk. Scrape the little leftover bits from the chops. Upon completion, toss oregano, coriander, and thyme in. Please ensure you are only simmering and not boiling the sauce.

5. Lastly, as the sauce thickens, turn the heat off and toss chops back into skillet. Combine all elements and add more pepper & salt if desired. Serve with veggies or a fresh salad.

Savory Idea #7: Filet & Cheese Supreme

Number of people served: 3 or 4

Time you'll need: 31 to 36 minutes

Calories: 211

Fats: 17.4 g

Proteins: 11.9 g

Carbs: 2.25 g

**What you'll require:**

- Paprika (4.5 g)
- Fish Fillet (225 g)
- Parsley (flakes, 7.5 g)
- Pepper (black, 4.5 g)
- Oil (Olive, 18.5 g)
- Cheese (Parmesan, 45 g)

**What you need to do:**

1. First, heat up the oven to approximately 180 degrees Celsius.
2. Now, get mixing container for the pepper (black), paprika, cheese (Parmesan), and parsley.
3. Then, cover filets with the spice mix. Add oil (olive) and then rollup the mixture ensuring an even coating.
4. Once the fish is ready, set the filets on to tray and place it into the oven for roughly fourteen to seventeen minutes.
5. Lastly, double-check fish is thoroughly cooked and place cheese on top to create a crust. Let sit for a few moments, until cheese is crispy, remove, and serve. Enjoy with veggies or low-carb brown rice.

Savory Idea #8: Quick and Easy Low-carb Chips

Number of people served: 4

Time you'll need: 28 to 34 minutes

Calories: 91.7

Fats: 8.1 g

Proteins: 3.2 g

Carbs: 2.8 g

**What you'll require:**

- Salt (as preferred)
- Pepper (as preferred)
- Bacon (slices, eight)
- Oil (Olive, 18.5 g)

**What you need to do:**

1. First, set up an oven to approximately 180 degrees Celsius.
2. Next, grease a tray with oil (olive) or your choice of grease. Then, break up the bacon into small, bite-sized pieces.
3. After, season with pepper & salt as per your taste.
4. Then, throw into the oven for roughly eighteen to twenty-one minutes. Remove and let cool.
5. Once cool to touch, take bits and put into a skillet, or pan, over medium fire. This process usually takes about four to six minutes. Remove from fire and serve as chips. You can serve with a low-fat, low-carb dip as an appetizer!

Savory Idea #9: Unbelievably Low-carb South Treat

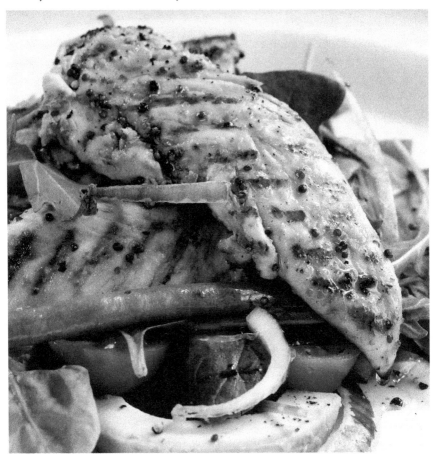

Number of people served: 3 to 4

Time you'll need: 29 to 32 minutes

Calories: 288

Fats: 22.3 g

Proteins: 18.9 g

Carbs: 2.7 g

**What you'll require:**

- Turkey Breast (roasted, 225 g, chopped)
- Cheese (Parmesan, 75 g)
- Cheddar Cheese (shredded, 225 g)
- White Cheddar Cheese (shredded, 225 g)

**What you need to do:**

1. First, set up an oven to approximately 180 degrees Celsius.
2. Next, take a mixing container and combine all cheeses. You can whisk or use an electric mixer. Then, take a spoonful of the mix and place onto baking sheet in a clump. Lay down as you would with cookies. Space clumps about one inch apart.
3. Upon filling sheet, throw into over for roughly seven to eight minutes. Please ensure that chips do not get burned. Chips are cooked thoroughly when edges turn light to a golden brown. Then, remove and let cool all the way.
4. Lastly, chop up turkey breast and serve chips with a low-sugar dip. Serve as a snack or entrée.

Savory Idea #10: Low-sugar Italian Snack Option

Number of people served: 4 to 6
Time you'll need: About 22 minutes

Calories: 226
Fats: 23.7 g
Proteins: 18.4 g
Carbs: 5.7 g

**What you'll require:**

- Mozzarella Cheese (shredded, 225 g)
- Pepper (as preferred)
- Seasoning (Italian, 14.5 g)
- Pepperoni (115 g, chopped)
- Garlic (powder, 8.5 g)
- Salt (as preferred)
- Additional choice: Marinara Sauce for Dipping

**What you need to do:**

1. First, set up an oven to approximately 180 degrees Celsius.
2. Next, take a small muffin tray and coat with spray (cooking). Leave to one side.
3. Then, in a mixing container, combine pepper & cheese, garlic (powder), salt, and seasoning (Italian). Mix cheese thoroughly and add in the seasoning. Place spoonful of mixture into the bottom of each space on tray.
4. After, top each space with pepperoni. Once ready, place into the oven for about eight to ten minutes. After this time, the cheese should be melted all the way through and light brown around the sides.
5. Lastly, remove, let cool, and serve with low-sugar sauce (marinara works best). Serve as a snack or side for a meat dish.

# Chapter 4: Gourmet Recipe Ideas

Gourmet Idea #1: Tasty Chicken and Veggie Pot

Number of people served: 4 to 6
Time you'll need: 26 to 32 minutes

Calories: 238
Fats: 10.9g
Proteins: 27.6g
Carbs: 2.7g

**What you'll require:**

- Broccoli (one bag, frozen)
- Chicken (115g, shredded)
- Garlic Powder (as preferred)
- Soup (Cream of Mushroom, one can)
- Pepper (as preferred)
- Cheese (Cheddar 221g)

**What you need to do:**

1. First, prepare the oven to approximately 185 degrees Celsius.
2. Then, in a mixing container, toss in the various elements you will be using (chicken, cheese, and spices)
3. Next, add in soup.
4. Then, place the mixture into a baking container and insert it into the oven.
5. After, let cook in the oven for about twenty-five to thirty minutes.
6. Lastly, ensure that the soup has been thoroughly cooked and cheese properly melted. Serve with a side of crispy veggies or almond breadsticks.

Gourmet Idea #2: Delicious Low-sugar Chicken Meal

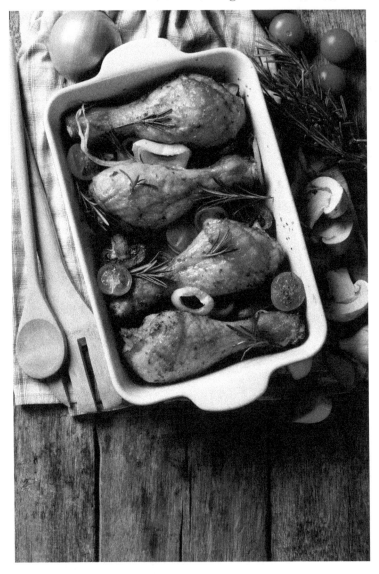

Number of people served: 4

Time you'll need: Approximately 30 minutes

Calories: 384

Fats: 21.1g

Proteins: 48.1g

Carbs: 3.2g

**What you'll require:**

- Cream (Sour, 221 g)
- Salt (9.5 g)
- Chicken (Breast, 1kg, no bone)
- Garlic (Powder, 14.5g)
- Pepper (4.5 g)
- Cheese (Parmesan, 165g, grated)

**What you need to do:**

1. First, prepare the oven to approximately 185 degrees Celsius.
2. Next, prepare a baking container with grease (or your choice such as spray)
3. After, in a mixing tray, add sour cream and a cup of cheese (Parmesan)
4. Then, place the chicken (breast) into the tray while spreading the mix atop each piece. Also, cover lightly with leftover cheese.
5. After that, insert the tray into the oven. Let it sit there for about twenty-seven to twenty-nine minutes.
6. Lastly, remove once thoroughly cooked and serve with your favorite low-carb side.

Gourmet Idea #3: Italian Chicken Dinner Delight

Number of people served: 2 to 4

Time you'll need: Approximately 25 minutes

Calories: 581

Fats: 41.1g

Proteins: 48.2g

Carbs: 6.1g

**What you'll require:**

- Garlic (Cloves, two, Minced)
- Tomatoes (Sun-dried, 65g)
- Spinach (221g, Chopped)
- Chicken (Breast, four)
- Paprika (8.5g)
- Cream (Heavy, 221 g)
- Garlic (Powder, 8.5g)
- Butter (14.5 g)
- Salt (8.5g)

**What you need to do:**

1. First, combine garlic (powder), paprika, and salt into mixing container. Upon completion, use this mixture to coat chicken lightly.

2. Next, fire up a skillet, or pan, and throw in two spoonfuls of butter at the base. Let the butter melt. After this, add in properly seasoned

chicken and let cook thoroughly. This would take about five minutes per side. Please ensure chicken is cooked all the way through. Remove and place to one side.

3. Then, add in the rest of the elements: tomatoes, cream, and tomatoes. It will take about three minutes on low fire for the mix to thicken. After, toss in spinach and mix up everything for four more minutes.

4. Lastly, throw the chicken back into the mix so that all flavors can combine. Ensure that chicken is properly cooked and season further if needed. Serve with a side of veggies, zucchini pasta, or low-carb couscous.

Gourmet Idea #4: Yummy Lemon Beef Surprise
Number of people served: 4
Time you'll need: Approximately three hours

Calories: 507
Fats: 35.1g
Proteins: 44.8g
Carbs: 3.1g

**What you'll require:**

- Pepper (4.5g)
- Lemon (one)
- Garlic (Cloves, four, Crushed)
- Salt (4.5 g)
- Beef (one kg, Cubed)
- Parsley (26g, Minced)

**What you need to do:**

1. First, prepare the oven to approximately 167 degrees Celsius.
2. Then, prepare a baking container with foil lining.
3. Next, get a mixing container and cover beef (cubed) with juice (lemon), some zest (lemon), salt, and garlic as preferred. Once it is ready to taste, fold over foil to create a small package.
4. Then, when the package is ready, insert into the middle section of the oven and let sit for roughly three hours. This longer cooking time is intended to let the meat soften to its best point.
5. Lastly, remove the package and let sit for about five or six minutes. Cover meat with more juice (lemon) and sprinkle parsley on top. Serve with your favorite low-carb side.

## Gourmet Idea #5: Gourmet Sirloin Option

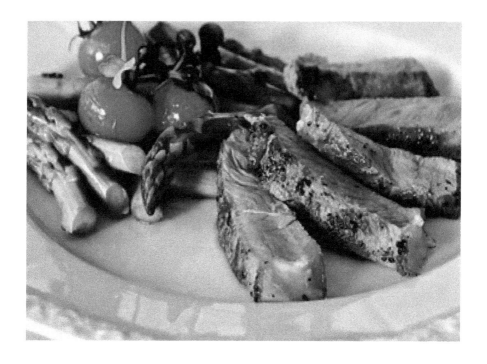

Number of people served: 3 to 4

Time you'll need: 25 to 30 minutes

Calories: 389

Fats: 18.9g

Proteins: 47.1g

Carbs: 2.3g

**What you'll require:**

- Garlic (Cloves, four, Crushed)
- Oil (Olive, 12g)
- Pepper & salt (as preferred)
- Steak (Sirloin, 945g, Cubed)
- Butter (14.5 g)

**What you need to do:**

1. First, get an iron skillet or pan and place it on high heat and place oil (olive).
2. Next, add in pepper & salt to the steak as per your preference.
3. Once the steak has been seasoned according to your preference, place it in the hot skillet, or pan, with hot oil. Let the steak in the hot oil for about four minutes on each side. Turnover twice. Then remove. After, using the same skillet, or pan, toss in butter and garlic. Please ensure to move constantly, so the mix doesn't get burnt.
4. When the garlic is light or golden brown. Place meat for another couple of minutes on each side. Let simmer until the flavors are combined. Serve with your favorite side.

Gourmet Idea #6: Unbelievably Low-sugar Surprise

Number of people served: 4 to 6

Time you'll need: Approximately 20 minutes

Calories: 171

Fats: 11.8g

Proteins: 14.6g

Carbs: 2.9g

**What you'll require:**

- Cheese (Mozzarella, 100g, Shredded)
- Cheese (Parmesan, 75g, Grated)
- Cheddar Cheese (Shredded, 75g)
- Eggs (two)
- Ham (221g, Diced)

**What you need to do:**

1. First, set up oven to 185 degrees Celsius.
2. Next, get a mixing container so you can combine egg and the various types of cheeses (shredded). After thoroughly mixing, toss in ham (diced) and continue combining until mixture is evenly distributed.
3. After, get a baking container so it can be greased (your choice of grease).
4. Now, separate mixture into eight round balls or rolls.
5. Then, insert the baking container into the oven for approximately twenty minutes. The rolls will be ready once the cheese has melted, and a golden-brown crust has formed.
6. Lastly, remove the dish and allow it to cool. Serve with chicken or any other meat of your choice.

Gourmet Idea #7: Low-carb Salmon Delight

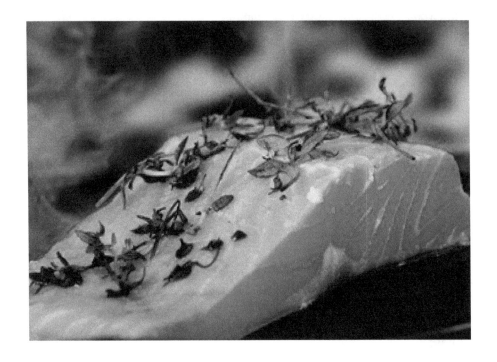

Number of people served: 3 to 4

Time you'll need: 18 to 24 minutes

Calories: 276

Fats: 19.1g

Proteins: 24.5g

Carbs: 3.7g

**What you'll require:**

- Rosemary (Fresh, two Springs)
- Lemon (55 g)
- Pepper (as preferred)
- Garlic (Cloves, three)
- Salt (4.5 g)
- Salmon (Filets, four)
- Butter (Unsalted, 8.5g)

**What you need to do:**

1. First, start out by setting the oven to 202 degrees Celsius.
2. Next, line baking container with a sheet of paper (parchment) and set to the side.
3. Then, rinse out filets (salmon) and pat down to try. Upon completion, place on the baking container with the skin facing down.
4. After, take some soft butter to cover the top of the filer. Also, add in some pepper & salt according to your liking.
5. Now, add the spices (rosemary) and the garlic. Cover the filet and insert it into the oven for roughly thirteen to sixteen minutes.
6. Lastly, remove the filet when thoroughly cooked. Add some juice (lemon) to add a tangy zest. Serve with a side of veggies for a nutritious meal.

Gourmet Idea #8: Shrimp-Avocado Treat

Number of people served: 4

Time you'll need: 30 to 35 minutes

Calories: 539

Fats: 45.2g

Proteins: 25.8g

Carbs: 6.1g

**What you'll require:**

- Onion (62.5g)
- Cooked shrimp (455g, Chopped)
- Eggs (two)
- Seasoning (Seafood, 4.5g)
- Juice (Lemon, 8.5g)
- Parsley (Fresh, 14.5g)
- Crab (Cooked 125g)
- Avocados (four)
- Cheese (Cheddar, 221 g, Shredded)

**What you need to do:**

1. First, start out by setting the oven to 177 degrees Celsius.
2. Then, in a mixing container, combine the ingredients: eggs, seasoning (seafood), juice (lemon), onion (chopped), cheese (cheddar), parsley, shrimp, and crab.
3. Next, as the stuffing is completed, cut up avocados in half and remove the pit. Then replace the pit with the stuffing.
4. Lastly, insert the avocados in the oven for roughly twenty-seven minutes. Remove from oven and serve with almond breadsticks.

Gourmet Idea #9: Gourmet Hot Pot Surprise

Number of people served: 4 to 6
Time you'll need: Approximately 45 minutes

Calories: 287
Fats: 20.8g
Proteins: 21.9g
Carbs: 4.8g

**What you'll require:**

- Cheese (Swiss, 70g, Shredded)
- Pepper (as preferred)
- Garlic (Cloves, four, Minced)
- Fish (Filet, your choice, 455g)
- Shrimp (455g)
- Cream (Heavy, 87g)
- Paprika (as preferred)
- Salt (as preferred)

**What you need to do:**

1. First, start out by setting the oven to 191 degrees Celsius.

2. Next, prepare a baking container with grease (your choice).

3. Then, cut the filet (fish) into small to medium-sized pieces and place them on the bottom of the baking container. Then, place a layer of shrimp on top of the fish. Add pepper & salt as per your liking.

4. After, when you have everything layered, add in garlic and heavy cream to cover. Upon liberally covering, add cheese (Swiss) on top. Add a touch of paprika for that tangy edge.

5. Now, insert into the oven for roughly sixteen to eighteen minutes. Check often to make sure it does not overcook.

6. Lastly, serve with almond bread!

Gourmet Idea #10: Low-carb Tuna Wraps Treat

Number of people served: 4

Time you'll need: About 10 minutes

Calories: 109

Fats: 5.7g

Proteins: 7.8g

Carbs: 7.1g

**What you'll require:**

- Yogurt (Greek, 50g)
- Wrap (Wheat, four)
- Bell Pepper (Red, 25g, Diced)
- Spinach (45g)
- Celery (65g, Diced)
- Tuna (one can)

**What you need to do:**

1. First, drain liquid from the can, and place tuna into a mixing container. Once this is in place, add in the red bell pepper, celery, and the Greek yogurt. Combine elements together well, so the vegetables and tuna are combined thoroughly.
2. Next, you are going to want to place the mixture into the middle of the whole-wheat wraps and top off with the spinach.
3. Serve with veggie chips and lemonade for a refreshing brunch treat.

# Chapter 5: Quick and Easy Recipe Ideas

Quick and Easy Idea #1: Quick and Easy Veggie Treat

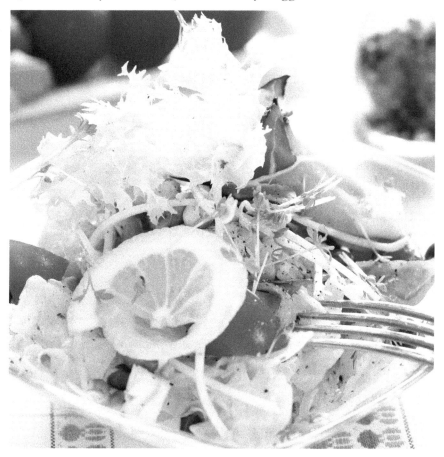

Number of people served: 4

Time you'll need: 35 to 40 minutes

Calories: 51

Fats: 3.1 g

Proteins: 4.5 g

Carbs: 2.3 g

**What you'll require:**

- Egg (whites, two)
- Spinach (221g, chopped)
- Eggs (whole, two)
- Pepper (Bell, one)
- Salsa (14.5g)
- Onion (35g, chopped)
- Pepper & salt (as preferred)

**What you need to do:**

1. First, place the pan over medium fire. Once it is warm, throw in some oil (olive) and start by placing spinach and onion until reaching consistency to your preference. Season with pepper plus salt. Add more salsa if you wish.

2. Next, let your vegetables cook, cut up a bell pepper in two slices to create a small bowl. Upon completion, add the spinach mix to the pepper bowls and the open an egg on top.

3. Then, insert into the oven for about 25 to 28 minutes. Make sure to see that egg is thoroughly prepared.

4. Lastly, serve as a side to your favorite meat dish.

Quick and Easy Idea #2: Spicy Egg and Veggie Dash

Number of people served: 12

Time you'll need: 30 to 35 minutes

Calories: 242

Fats: 21.7 g

Proteins: 10.2 g

Carbs: 1.1 g

**What you'll require:**

- Bacon (in strips, 11)
- Onion (Powder, 4.5g)
- Garlic (Powder, 4.5g)
- Cheese (cream, 95g)
- Pepper & salt (as preferred)
- Eggs (8)
- Peppers (Jalapeno, four, Chopped)
- Cheese (Cheddar, 121 g)

**What you need to do:**

1. First, fire up the oven to 165 degrees Celsius.
2. Then, fire up bacon until crispy.
3. Next, in another container, mix up chopped jalapenos, eggs, cheese (cream), and seasoning. Toss in leftover bacon grease.

4. Then, take a muffin baking container and fill the edge of each space with bacon. Upon completion, pour in the mix down the middle of each space. Fill up to about 2/3 of the way. This is important as eggs will rise.

5. After, add some cheese (cheddar) and some jalapeno to provide spice. Insert into the oven and let cook for about 22 to 24 minutes. These will be ready when eggs are thoroughly done and fluffy.

6. Lastly, remove and serve as a snack or an appetizer.

Quick and Easy Idea #3: Low-sugar Hot Cake Surprise

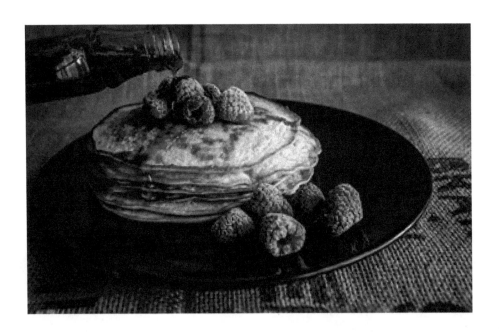

Number of people served: 10

Time you'll need: Approximately 20 minutes

Calories: 133

Fats: 11.8 g

Proteins: 5.3 g

Carbs: 1.9 g

**What you'll require:**

- Flour (Almond, 221 g)
- Eggs (4)
- Milk (Almond, Non-sugar, 36.5g)
- Extract (Vanilla, 7.5g)
- Baking Powder (4.7g)
- Oil (Olive, 18.5g)

**What you need to do:**

1. First, in a mixing container, mix up baking powder, extract (vanilla), milk (almond), flour (almond), and eggs. Please ensure all clumps are removed.
2. Next, use a tablespoon to place mixture into pan or skillet. Prepare these as you would regular pancakes.
3. Last, top with butter or non-sugar syrup.

## Quick and Easy Idea #4: Cheesy Veggie Bites

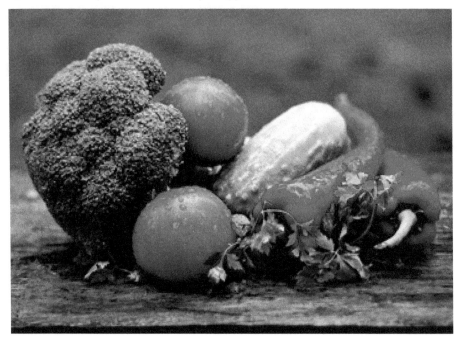

Number of people served: 4

Time you'll need: Approximately 30 minutes

Calories: 161

Fats: 11.6 g

Proteins: 11.4 g

Carbs: 5.1 g

**What you'll require:**

- Flour (Almond, 36.5g)
- Onion (36.5g, minced)

- Seasoning (Mexican, 8.5g)
- Mozzarella (221g, shredded)
- Broccoli (225g)
- Salt (as preferred)
- Garlic (clove, one, minced)
- Cilantro (17.5g)
- Egg (one)
- Pepper (as preferred)

**What you need to do:**

1. First, set up 201 degrees Celsius.
2. Next, prepare a baking container by lining with parchment paper.
3. Then, steam broccoli in a pot (5 minutes) or microwave (1-2 minutes). Tenderize broccoli to make chopping easier.
4. After, cut up broccoli into small chunks. Throw everything into mixing container (parsley, cheese, flour, egg, and spices). Mix up thoroughly until evenly distributed.
5. Now, roll up into a small ball and distribute evenly throughout the baking container.
6. Once completed, cover with some oil (olive) and insert it into the oven for about 26 to 28 minutes.
7. Lastly, serve with low-carb dip as a snack.

Quick and Easy Idea #5: Low-carb Pudding Dee-light

Number of people served: 4

Time you'll need: 18 to 20 minutes

Calories: 132

Fats: 12.1g

Proteins: 13.8g

Carbs: 1.4g

## What you'll require:

- Coconut (125g, shredded)
- Almonds (221g, chopped)
- Chia seed (221g)
- Milk (almond, 225g)

## What you need to do:

1. First, measure out all of the fixings and add to the Instant Pot, stirring well.
2. Then, secure the lid and select the high setting (2-5 minutes)
3. Lastly, quick release the pressure and place the pudding into four serving glasses.

Quick and Easy Idea #6: Tangy Egg Salad

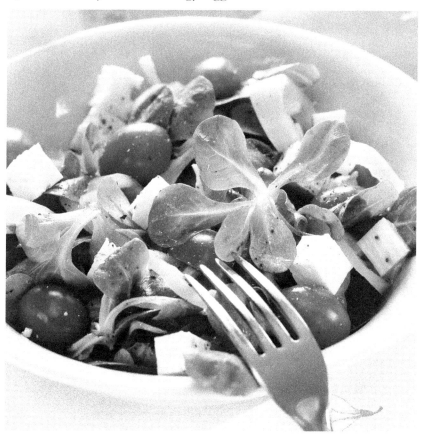

Number of people served: 4 to 5

Time you'll need: 26 to 32 minutes

Calories: 314

Fats: 25.7g

Proteins: 15.4g

Carbs: 1.4g

**What you'll require:**

- Bacon (strips, five, raw)
- Paprika (smoked, 14.5)
- Eggs (large, 10)
- Onion (green, 36.5g)
- Mayonnaise (125g)
- Mustard (Dijon, 45g)
- Pepper & salt (as preferred)

Also required: 6-7-inch baking container

**What you need to do:**

1. First, grease up all sides of the pan inside of pot on the trivet. Toss one cup of cold water in the bottom of the Instant Pot and add the steam rack.
2. Next, open up eggs in a pan.
3. Then, insert pan on rack. Secure the lid and set the timer for 6 minutes (high-pressure). Natural release the pressure to remove pan.
4. After, remove any moisture. Flip pan over on a wooden cutting board for egg loaf to release. Cut up and place it into a mixing dish.
5. Now, clean the Instant Pot container and choose the sauté function (medium fire). Prepare bacon till crispy.
6. After that, add in chopped eggs with mustard, mayo, paprika, pepper, and salt. Top with green onion.
7. Lastly, serve as a side with your favorite meat dish.

Quick and Easy Idea #7: Cheesy Egg Cups

Number of people served: 4
Time you'll need: 12 to 16 minutes

Calories: 117
Fats: 8.8g
Proteins: 8.7g
Carbs: 1.8g

**What you'll require:**

- Eggs (four)
- Cheese (Cheddar, 125g, shredded)
- Veggies (diced, your choice, veggies tomatoes, mushrooms, and/or peppers, 221g)
- Milk (low-fat, non-sugar, 221g)
- Pepper & salt (as preferred)
- Cilantro (chopped, 125g)

**What you'll require for the Topping:**

- Cheese (shredded, your choice, 221g)

**Also Required:**

1. Jars (medium, four)
2. Water (0.5L)

**What you need to do:**

1. First, whisk up cheese, veggies, pepper, eggs, milk (low-fat), salt, and cilantro.
1. Next, combine the mix into each jar. Tighten lids (not too tight) to keep water from entering the egg mix.
2. Then, arrange the trivet in the Instant Pot and add the water. Arrange the jars on the trivet and set the timer for 5 minutes (high pressure). When done, quick release the pressure, and top with the rest of the cheese (½ cup).
3. Lastly, broil if you like for 2 to 4 minutes till the cheese is browned to your preference.

Quick and Easy Idea #8: Asparagus Appetizer/Side Salad

Number of people served: 4 to 6

Time you'll need: 18 to 22 minutes

Calories: 221

Fats: 8.6g

Proteins: 15.7g

Carbs: 8.1g

**What you'll require:**

- Red potatoes (small, 455g)
- Asparagus (fresh, trimmed and chopped lengthwise)
- Tuna (2 tins)
- Olives (Greek, 125g, pit removed)
- Dressing (Italian, low sugar, 45g)

**What you need to do:**

1. First, chop potatoes and let soak in water for about 5 minutes to let starch drain.
2. Next, put water in the pot, about 2 inches, and heat up to a boiling point. Throw in chopped potatoes to cook for about 12 to 14 minutes.
3. Then, in the remaining 2 to 4 minutes of cooking potatoes, add asparagus to the water.
4. After, turn off the heat, remove water from asparagus and potatoes and then place it into ice water.
5. Lastly, serve with tuna and olives as an appetizer or side for a chicken or fish dish.

## Quick and Easy Idea #9: Low-carb Pork Treat

Number of people served: 4 to 6
Time you'll need: 18 to 22 minutes

Calories: 221
Fats: 8.6g
Proteins: 15.7g
Carbs: 8.1g

**What you'll require:**

- Pork (tenderloin, 455g)
- Salt (14.5g)
- Pepper (18.5g)
- Oil (Olive, 75g)
- Cider (apple, 95g)
- Syrup (maple, non-sugar, 25g)
- Vinegar (apple cider)

**What you need to do:**

1. First, set up your oven to 190 degrees Celsius.
2. Next, cut up tenderloin into two pieces or to fit in the pan or skillet you are using. Transfer into another container.
3. Then, put oil in pan, or skillet, and then fire up for about 6 to 8 minutes. Toss in vinegar, syrup, and cider while adding pepper until boiling point. Make sure to remove bits stuck to the bottom.
4. After, throw in meat. Prepare thoroughly until the mixture is reduced to glazed texture.
5. Lastly, remove and serve while adding sauce for glazing. Serve with a side of veggies.

Quick and Easy Idea #10: Easy Fish Delight

Number of people served: 4 to 6    Time you'll need: 18 to 22 minutes

Calories: 257

Fats: 8.8g

Proteins: 25.7g

Carbs: 9.2g

**What you'll require:**

- Breadcrumbs (low-carb, 56g)
- Oil (Olive, 45g)
- Dill (fresh, 45g, snipped)
- Salt (10.5g)
- Pepper (5g)
- Filet (tilapia or salmon, 50g per filet)
- Juice (lemon, 25g)
- Lemon (wedges)

**What you need to do:**

1. First, set up the oven to 186 degrees Celsius. Add the pepper, oil (olive), dill (fresh), salt, and juice (lemon).
2. Next, add filet (fish of your choice) into a baking container which has been previously coated with grease. Add breadcrumbs on top of fish patting down to so they stick. Coat both sides.
3. Then, let sit in the oven until fish is tender, roughly for 12 to 14 minutes.
4. Lastly, serve with veggies and add lemon wedges on top.

# Chapter 6: Low-Carb Recipe Ideas

Low-Carb Recipe Idea #1: Balsamic Roast Delight

Number of people served: 4 to 6

Time you'll need: 35 to 40 minutes

Calories: 51

Fats: 3.1 g

Proteins: 4.5 g

Carbs: 2.3 g

**What you'll require:**

- Chuck roast (one, no bone, 1.5kg)

- Onion (chopped, 55g)

- Water (0.5L)

- Ground pepper (black, 14.5g)

- Garlic (powder, 14.5g)

- Salt (kosher, 14.5g)

- Vinegar (balsamic, 14.5g)

- Xanthan gum (25g)

**For Garnishing:**

- Fresh parsley (chopped, 20g)

**What you need to do:**

1. First, combine the garlic powder, salt, and pepper and spread on the meat to prepare the seasoning.

2. Next, utilize the skillet to sear the meat. Add in the vinegar and deglaze the skillet, or pan, while you let cook for another couple of minutes.

3. Then, toss in onion into a pot along with (two cups) boiling water into the mixture. Cover with a top and allow simmer for thirty to forty minutes on medium-low heat.

4. After, remove meat from pot and add to a cutting surface. Shred up into chunks and throw away any fat and/or bones.

5. Now, add in the xanthan gum to the broth and mix up briskly. Place the thoroughly cooked meat back into the pan to heat up.

6. Lastly, serve with a favorite side dish.

Low-Carb Recipe Idea #2: Burger Calzone Treat

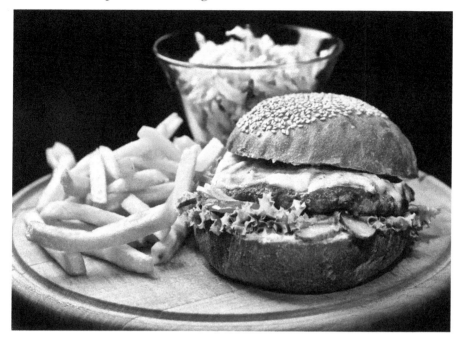

Number of people served: 6
Time you'll need: 25 to 30 minutes

Calories: 400
Fats: 25.1g
Proteins: 24.5 g
Carbs: 2.6 g

**What you'll require:**

- Mayonnaise (45g)
- Onion (yellow, one diced)
- Beef (ground, 750g, lean)
- Cheese (cheddar, 75g, shredded)
- Flour (Almond, 95g)
- Cheese (Mozzarella, 75g, shredded)
- Egg (one)

- Bacon (4 thin strips)
- Dill pickle (4 spears)
- Cheese (cream, 95g)

**What you need to do:**

1. First, program the oven to 185 degrees Celsius. Set up a baking container with parchment paper.

2. Next, chop up pickles into lengthy spears. Set to one side when completed.

3. Then, to prepare the crust, combine half of the cream cheese and the mozzarella. Insert into microwave 30 seconds. Upon melting, add egg and almond flour to prepare the dough. Set aside.

4. After, set the beef to fire on the stove using a medium temp setting.

5. Now, cook bacon (microwave for approximately four minutes or on the stovetop with pan or skillet). Upon cooling, break up into bits.

6. Now, dice up an onion and toss into the beef to cook until tenderized. Throw in bacon, pickle bits, cheddar cheese, the rest of the cream cheese, and mayonnaise. Move briskly.

7. After that, roll the dough into a prepared baking container. Place the mixture into the middle of the container. Fold up ends and side to create the calzone.

8. Lastly, insert into until brown or about 12 to 14 minutes. Let it rest for 10 minutes before cutting up.

Low-Carb Recipe Idea #3: Steak Skillet Nacho

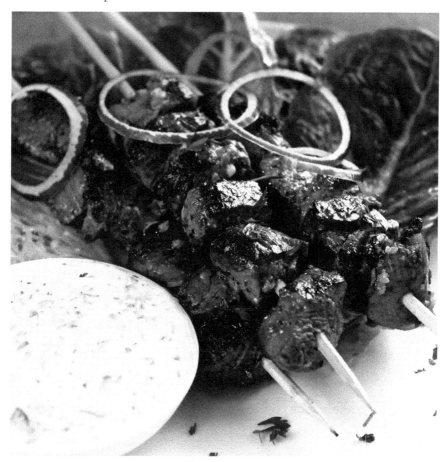

Number of people served: 3 to 4

Time you'll need: 26 to 33 minutes

Calories: 376

Fats: 31.5g

Proteins: 19.4g

Carbs: 6.1 g

## What you'll require:

- Cheese (Cheddar, 75g)

- Coconut oil (45g)

- Butter (15g)

- Beef (Steak, round tip, 1kg)

- Cauliflower (750g)

- Turmeric (15g)

- Chili (powder, 15g)

- Cheese (Monterey Jack, 75g)

**For Garnishing:**

- Sour cream (25g)

- Jalapeno (canned, 20g, slices)

- Avocado (105g)

**What you need to do:**

1. First, set up oven temp to 176 degrees Celsius.
2. Next, prepare the cauliflower into chip-like shapes.
3. After, combine the chili powder, turmeric, and coconut oil in a mixing container.
4. Then, throw in cauliflower and add it to a container. Set the timer for 18 to 24 minutes.
5. Now, over a med-high fire in a cast iron pan, place butter. Fire up until both sides are thoroughly done, flipping only one time. Let it sit for six to nine minutes. Slice up thinly and add in some pepper and salt to the meat.
6. After that, move the florets to the pan and add in the steak bits. Top it off with the cheese and bake six to nine more minutes.
7. Lastly, serve with your favorite side of veggies.

Low-Carb Recipe Idea #4: Portobello Burger Meal

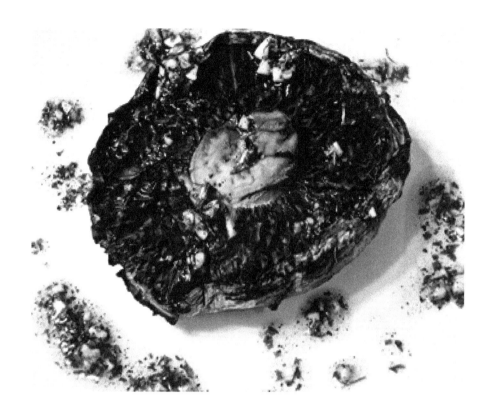

Number of people served: 4

Time you'll need: 22 to 27 minutes

Calories: 327

Fats: 23.1g

Proteins:19.4g

Carbs: 6.1 g

**What you'll require:**

- Mushroom (Portobello, 6 caps)

- Beef (ground, 455g, lean)

- Pepper (Black, 6g, ground)

- Worcestershire sauce (14.5g)

- Salt (pink or kosher, 12g)

- Cheese (cheddar, 56g or 6 slices)

- Oil (avocado, 12g)

**What you need to do:**

1. First, remove the stem, rinse, and dab dry the mushrooms.

2. Then, combine the salt, pepper, beef, and Worcestershire sauce in a mixing container. Shape into patties.

3. After, fire up the oil (medium fire). Let caps simmer about four to five minutes on each side.

4. Next, move the mushrooms to a bowl, utilizing the same pan, prepare the patties for six minutes, turn, and prepare another six minutes until ready.

5. Now, combine the cheese to the patties and cover for about a minute to melt the cheese.

6. Lastly, add a mushroom cap to burgers along with the desired garnish to serve.

Low-Carb Recipe Idea #5: Low-carb Super Chili

Number of people served: 4
Time you'll need: 20 to 24 minutes

Calories: 319
Fats: 24.1g
Proteins:39.2g
Carbs: 3.4g

## What you'll require for the Chili:

- Stock (beef or chicken, 25g)
- Steak (1kg, cubed into 1-inch cubes)
- Leeks (sliced, 25g)
- Cumin (4g)
- Cayenne pepper (ground, 4g)
- Pepper (black, 4g)
- Salt (4g)
- Whole tomatoes (canned with juices, 221g)
- Chili powder (2.5g)

## Additional Toppings:

- Cheese (cheddar, 221g, shredded)
- Sour cream (95g)
- Cilantro (fresh, 25g, chopped)
- Avocado (one half, sliced or cubed)

## What you need to do:

1. First, toss all of the fixings into the cooker - except the toppings.

2. Then, use the cooker's high setting for about six hours.

3. Lastly, serve and add the toppings.

Low-Carb Recipe Idea #6: "You won't believe it's low-carb" Chicken Parmesan

Number of people served: 2 to 4

Time you'll need: 34 to 40 minutes

Calories: 586

Fats: 31.4g

Proteins:55.5g

Carbs: 2.7g

## What you'll require:

- Rinds (pork, 221g)
- Sauce (Marinara, 45g)
- Chicken (breast, 455g)
- Cheese (parmesan, 56g)
- Garlic (powder, 12g)
- Pepper & salt (as preferred)
- Egg (one)
- Cheese (Mozzarella, 125g, shredded)
- Oregano (12g)

## What you need to do:

1. First, set up an oven temp setting of 165 degrees Celsius.
2. Next, utilize a food processor to mash rinds and cheese (parmesan). Add them to a mixing container.

3. After, pound chicken breasts until they are about one-half inch thick. Whisk up egg and dip chicken in for the egg wash. Place the chicken into crumbs.

4. Then, distribute the breasts on a lightly greased baking container evenly. Add in seasonings and insert them into the oven for approximately 23 to 26 minutes.

5. Now, cover with the marinara sauce over each serving. Top with the mozzarella and bake for 12 to 14 minutes.

6. Lastly, serve with a bed of spinach.

Low-Carb Recipe Idea #7: Tangy Coconut Chicken

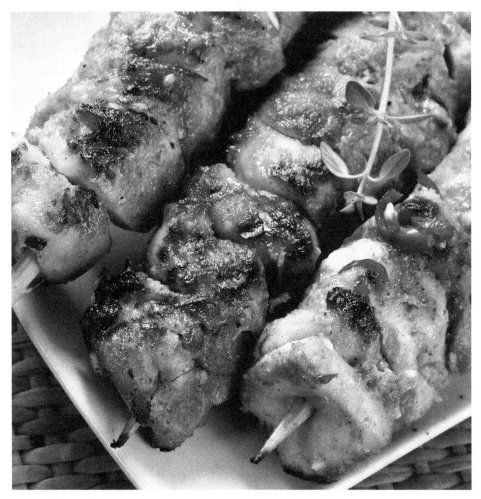

Number of people served: 4 to 5
Time you'll need: 25 to 28 minutes

Calories: 492
Fats: 39.7g
Proteins:28.9g
Carbs: 2.3g

## What you'll require for the Tenders:

- Egg (large, one)
- Onion (powder, 8.5g)
- Curry (powder, 18.5g)
- Pork rinds (Crumbled, 125g)
- Chicken (thighs, 1kg, no bone or skin, about 6 to 8 pieces)
- Coriander (14.5g)
- Coconut (shredded, 95g, unsweetened)
- Garlic (powder, 8.5g)
- Pepper & salt (as preferred)

**What you'll require for spicy and sweet mango sauce dip:**

- Sour cream (25g)
- Ginger (ground, 14.5g)
- Mango extract (15g)
- Mayonnaise (25g)
- Sugar-free ketchup(25g)
- Cayenne pepper (14g)
- Liquid stevia (7 to 8 drops)
- Garlic (powder, 8.5g)
- Red pepper (flakes, 5g)

**What you need to do:**

1. First, program oven to 185 degrees Celsius.
2. Then, whisk the eggs and debone the thighs. Slice them into strips (skins on).
3. Next, add the spices, coconut, and pork rinds to a zipper-type bag. Add the chicken, shake, and place on a wire rack. Bake for about 14 minutes. Flip them over and continue baking for another 18 minutes.
4. Lastly, combine the sauce components and stir well. Serve with your favorite side of veggies or salad.

Low-Carb Recipe Idea #8: Slow cook Chicken Casserole

Number of people served: 3 to 4

Time you'll need: 35 to 45 minutes

Calories: 224

Fats: 9.4g

Proteins:30.4g

Carbs: 5.7g

**What you'll require:**

- Chicken breasts (two in cubes)
- Bay leaf (one)
- Cheese (Mozzarella, 221g, shredded)
- Tomato sauce (256g or one tine)
- Seasoning (Italian, 14.5g)
- Salt (5.5g)
- Pepper (4g)
- Optional: slow cooker (2-quart)

**What you need to do:**

1. First, remove the bones from the chicken and chop it into cubes. Add them to the slow cooker.
2. Next, pour in the sauce over the chicken and add the spices. Stir and cook on the low setting for thirty to forty minutes.
3. Lastly, serve with the cheese as a topping.

Low-Carb Recipe Idea #9: Low-carb Roll Up Treat

Number of people served: 2 to 4
Time you'll need: 15 to 20 minutes

Calories: 191
Fats: 7.9g
Proteins:15.6g
Carbs: 1.9g

## What you'll require:

- Eggs (large, 6)
- Milk (221g)
- Garlic (powder, 14.5g)
- Salt (kosher, 9.5g)
- Pepper (Black, 9.5g, freshly ground)
- Butter (11g)
- Chives (chopped, 5g)
- Bacon (slices, 12)
- Cheese (cheddar, 105g)

## What you need to do:

- First, in mixing container, whisk up eggs together along with milk and garlic (powder). Add in salt & pepper as preferred.
- Next, in skillet or pan, melt butter over medium fire. Toss in eggs and scramble for 2 to 4 minutes. Toss in chives.
- Then, on a cutting surface, cut up bacon slices. Place cheddar on the bottom and then toss in a bunch of eggs. Roll up very closely.
- Lastly, place rolls back into pan, or skillet with the seam facing down. Remove once crispy. Serve with whole-grain toast.

Low-Carb Recipe Idea #10: Cauliflower Cheese Surprise

Number of people served: 2 to 4

Time you'll need: 10 to 20 minutes

Calories: 164

Fats: 6.5g

Proteins: 16.3g

Carbs: 2.4g

## What you'll require:

- Cauliflower (one Head, about 256g)
- Eggs (two)
- Cheese (parmesan, 75g)
- Oregano (35g)
- Cheese (cheddar, 75g, shredded)

## What you need to do:

- First, cut up cauliflower into individual florets. Place them into a food processor until the texture appears similar to rice. You could also grate if you don't have a processor.
- Then, in a mixing container, combine cauliflower, eggs, cheese (parmesan), and the oregano. Mix up until even and add salt & pepper.
- After, fire up a skillet, or pan, over medium fire. Todd mixture into the pan. Pat down to form a patty. Exert pressure using a spatula. Cook for 4 to 6 minutes. Turn over and repeat on the other side.
- Lastly, sprinkle cheese until it is melted. Make "sandwiches" by putting two pieces together. Serve as a snack or side to your favorite meat dish.

# Chapter 7: 7-day Sample Low Sugar Diet Plan

In this chapter, we are presenting a 7-day sample plan to give you an idea of how you can put together a winning combination of healthy foods. Please bear in mind that this is only a guide. So, feel free to customize this plan as you get more experience and develop your own style.

| Week One | | | |
|---|---|---|---|
| Day / Meal | Breakfast | Lunch | Dinner |
| Monday | Fresh fruit bowl topped with granola and honey | Veggie and chicken club sandwich on whole wheat bread | Chicken and veggie casserole |
| Tuesday | Spicy breakfast burritos | Bean soup with croutons | Grilled salmon and veggies |
| Wednesday | Scrambled eggs, bacon and a slice of whole-grain toast | Mixed garden salad, fresh veggies, and grilled chicken | Sirloin and veggies surprise |
| Thursday | Low-sugar cereal with low-fat | Steak and potatoes with a | Chicken fajitas with mashed |

|  | dairy milk | side of crispy veggies | potatoes |
|---|---|---|---|
| **Friday** | Veggie cheesy bits | Grilled salmon, sautéed veggies with garlic whole wheat toast | Roast beef club sandwich with crispy plantain bits |
| **Saturday** | Low-sugar whole grain flapjacks | Spicy chicken fajita burritos | Veggie pizza with small salad |
| **Sunday** | Whole grain veggie breakfast wraps | Tangy Mexican bean bowl with guacamole | Chicken noodles and sautéed veggies |

# PART III

# Air Fryer Recipes

The air fryer is a new mode of cooking advertised as a guilt-free and healthy way of enjoying all your favorite foods. Air fryer cooking claims that it can lower the fat content of various well-known food items such as chicken wings, French fries, fish sticks, and others. But, how healthy is it to cook in an air fryer?

Air fryer is a trendy appliance in the kitchen today that is being used for making food items like pastries, meat, and potato chips. It functions by simply circulating the hot air all around the food for producing crispy and crunchy exterior. All those food items that are air-fried are believed to be great alternatives for the deep-fried food items. There is no need to submerge the food items in oil. Just brush some oil, and you are good to go. It has been found that air fryer can cut off the fat content by 75%. The main reason behind this is that they need less amount of fat in comparison to deep fryers. For example, most of the deep-fried food items will require three cups of oil. But, the same can be cooked in an air fryer with only one tbsp. of oil.

In case you are willing to trim some extra fat around your waistline, substituting deep-fried food items with air-fried food items is a great way to start. So, it can be said that air-fryer can help in promoting weight loss. Frying food can produce dangerous compounds such as acrylamide. Cooking food in an air fryer can help you cut down the acrylamide content in your cooking. I have included some tasty air fryer recipes in this chapter that can be made with minimal effort.

# Chapter 1: Chicken And Pork Recipes

Meat forms an essential part of most types of diet. Here are some chicken and pork recipes that can be made easily using an air fryer.

## Maple Chicken Thighs

Total Prep & Cooking Time: One hour and thirty-five minutes

Yields: Four servings

Nutrition Facts: Calories: 410 | Protein: 22.3g | Carbs: 47.9g | Fat: 12.3g | Fiber: 1.2g

**Ingredients**

- One cup of buttermilk
- One large egg
- Half cup of maple syrup
- One tsp. of garlic (granulated)
- Four chicken thighs

*For the dry mix:*

- Half cup of flour
- One-fourth cup of tapioca flour
- One tbsp. of salt

- One tsp. of each
  - Sweet paprika
  - Onion (granulated)
  - Honey powder
- Half tsp. of paprika (smoked)
- One-fourth tsp. of each
  - Garlic (granulated)
  - Cayenne powder
  - Black pepper (ground)

**Method:**

1. Mix maple syrup, buttermilk, egg, and one tsp. of granulated garlic in a bowl. Add the thighs of chicken and marinate them for one hour.

2. Mix tapioca flour, flour, sweet paprika, salt, smoked paprika, pepper, granulated onion, half tsp. of granulated garlic, cayenne, and honey powder in a bowl.

3. Preheat your air fryer at 190 degrees Celsius.

4. Drain the marinade. Add the thighs in the flour mixture. Placechicken thighs in the air fryer basket. Cook them for ten minutes. Flip the chicken thighs and cook again for ten minutes.

Buttermilk Chicken

Total Prep & Cooking Time: Thirty-five minutes

Yields: Four servings

Nutrition Facts: Calories: 331 | Protein: 23.2g | Carbs: 26.3g | Fat: 10.6g | Fiber: 0.8g

**Ingredients**

- One cup of buttermilk
- Half tsp. of each
  - Hot sauce
  - Garlic salt
  - Paprika
  - Oregano
  - Onion powder
- One-third cup of tapioca flour
- One-eighth tsp. of black pepper (ground)
- One large egg
- Half cup of flour
- Two tsps. of brown sugar
- One tsp. of garlic powder
- One-fourth tsp. of black pepper
- One pound of chicken thighs (skinless, boneless)

**Method:**

1. Take a shallow dish and mix hot sauce with buttermilk.

2. Combine garlic salt, tapioca flour, and one-eighth tsp. of black pepper. Mix well.

3. Beat the egg in a bowl.

4. Mix salt, flour, brown sugar, paprika, garlic powder, onion powder, one-fourth tsp. of black pepper, and oregano in a bowl. Combine well.

5. Dip the thighs of chicken in this order: mixture of buttermilk, mixture of tapioca flour, beaten egg, and flour mixture.

6. Preheat your air fryer at 190 degrees Celsius. Use parchment paper for lining the fryer basket.

7. Cook the chicken thighs for ten minutes. Flip the thighs and cook again for ten minutes.

## Cheddar-Stuffed BBQ Breasts of Chicken

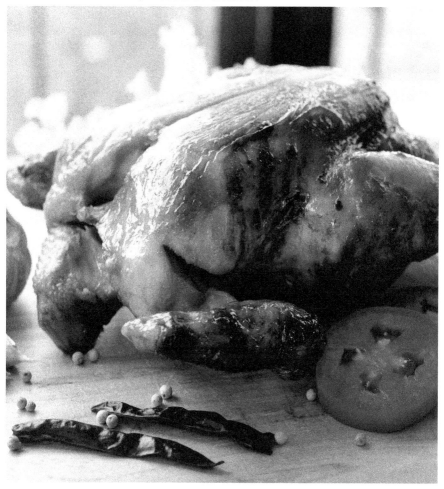

Total Prep & Cooking Time: Thirty-five minutes

Yields: Two servings

Nutrition Facts: Calories: 370 | Protein: 35.7g | Carbs: 11.7g | Fat: 17.7g | Fiber: 0.6g

## Ingredients

- Three bacon strips
- Two ounces of cheddar cheese (cubed)
- One-fourth cup of barbeque sauce
- Two chicken breasts (skinless)
- Pepper and salt

## Method:

1. Preheat your air fryer to 190 degrees Celsius. Cook a bacon strip in the air fryer for two minutes. Chop one strip of bacon. Use parchment paper for lining the fryer basket.

2. Mix cooked bacon, one tbsp. of barbeque sauce, and cheddar cheese.

3. Create a one-inch pouch at the top of the chicken breasts. Stuff the pouch with the mixture of bacon and cheese.

4. Wrap the bacon strips around the breasts of chicken. Use barbeque sauce for coating the chicken breasts.

5. Cook for ten minutes in the air fryer. Flip the chicken breasts and cook again for ten minutes.

## Buffalo Chicken

Total Prep & Cooking Time: Forty minutes

Yields: Four servings

Nutrition Facts: Calories: 230 | Protein: 30.2g | Carbs: 21.1g | Fat: 4.7g | Fiber: 1.9g

**Ingredients**

- Half cup of Greek yogurt
- One-fourth cup of egg substitute
- One tbsp. of each
  - Hot sauce
  - Sweet paprika
  - Cayenne pepper
  - Garlic pepper seasoning
- One tsp. of hot sauce
- One cup of bread crumbs
- One pound of chicken breast

**Method:**

1. Mix egg substitute, yogurt, and hot sauce in a mixing bowl.

2. Combine paprika, bread crumbs, cayenne pepper, and garlic pepper in a dish.

3. Dip the chicken breasts into the mixture of yogurt and coat in the mixture of bread crumbs.

4. Cook the chicken breasts in the air fryer for eight minutes. Flip the chicken breasts and cook again for five minutes.

## Breaded Pork Chops

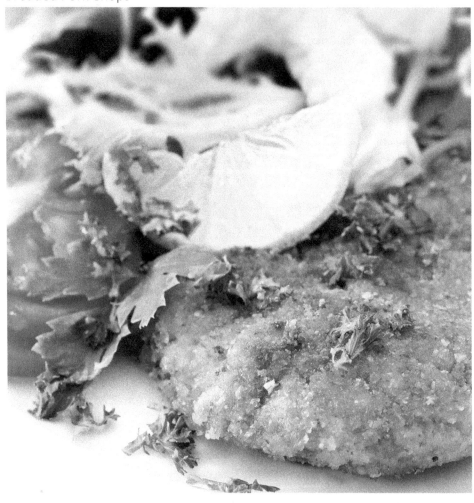

Total Prep & Cooking Time: Twenty minutes

Yields: Four servings

Nutrition Facts: Calories: 390 | Protein: 41.7g | Carbs: 10.3g | Fat: 17.1g | Fiber:

0.9g

**Ingredients**

- Four pork chops
- One tsp. of Cajun seasoning
- Two cups of garlic and cheese flavored croutons
- Two large eggs
- One cooking spray

**Method:**

1. Place the chops in a dish and season with the Cajun seasoning.

2. Add the croutons in a blender and pulse them.

3. Beat the eggs in a shallow dish.

4. Dip the pork chops into the beaten eggs and then coat in the blended croutons.

5. Use a cooking spray for misting the pork chops.

6. Cook the chops for five minutes. Flip the chops and cook again for five minutes.

## Pork Meatballs

Total Prep & Cooking Time: Thirty-five minutes

Yields: Twelve servings

Nutrition Facts: Calories: 120 | Protein: 8.4g | Carbs: 3.9g | Fat: 7.7g | Fiber: 0.3g

**Ingredients**

- Twelve ounces of pork (ground)
- Eight ounces of Italian sausage (ground)
- Half cup of panko bread crumbs
- One large egg
- One tsp. of each
  - Parsley (dried)
  - Salt
- Half tsp. of paprika

**Method:**

1. Combine sausage, pork, egg, bread crumbs, salt, paprika, and parsley in a bowl. Mix well. Make twelve meatballs using your hands.

2. Place the meatballs in the basket of the air fryer basket. Cook them for eight minutes. Shake the fryer basket and cook again for two minutes.

## Pork Jerky

Total Prep & Cooking Time: Eleven hours and ten minutes

Yields: Forty servings

Nutrition Facts: Calories: 56 | Protein: 4.4g | Carbs: 0.2g | Fat: 4.6g | Fiber: 0.1g

### Ingredients

- Two pounds of pork (ground)
- One tbsp. of each
  - Sesame oil
  - Sriracha
  - Soy sauce
  - Rice vinegar
- Half tsp. of each
  - Salt
  - Black pepper
  - Onion powder
  - Pink curing salt

### Method:

1. Mix pork, sriracha, sesame oil, soy sauce, vinegar, pepper, salt, onion powder, and curing salt in a bowl. Mix well and refrigerate for eight hours.

2. Use a jerky gun for making as many jerky sticks as possible.

3. Cook the jerky sticks in the fryer rack for one hour.

4. Flip the sticks and cook again for one hour.

5. Repeat step number four for three hours.

6. Transfer the sticks to a paper towel and soak excess fat.

7. Serve immediately, or you can store the sticks in the refrigerator for one month.

## Pork Skewers

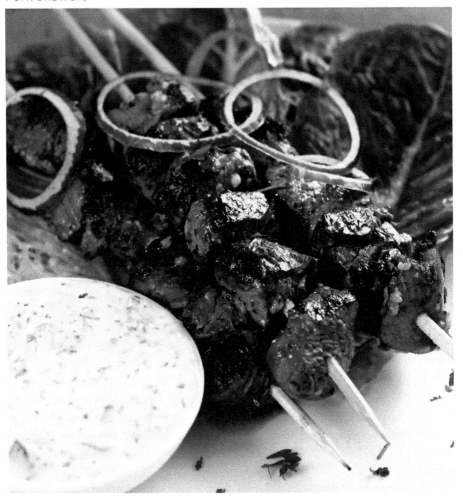

Total Prep & Cooking Time: Forty minutes

Yields: Forty servings

Nutrition Facts: Calories: 310 | Protein: 21g | Carbs: 30.6g | Fat: 9.2g | Fiber: 8.9g

**Ingredients**

- Two tbsps. of white sugar
- Five tsps. of onion powder
- Four tsps. of thyme (dried, crushed)
- One tbsp. of each
    - Black pepper (ground)
    - Allspice (ground)
    - Vegetable oil
    - Honey
    - Cilantro (chopped)
- Two tsps. of each
    - Salt
    - Cayenne pepper
- Three-fourth tsp. of nutmeg (ground)
- One-fourth tsp. of cloves (ground)
- One-fourth cup of coconut (shredded)
- One pound of pork tenderloin (cut in cubes of one inch)
- Four skewers
- One mango (peeled, chopped)
- Half a can of black beans (rinsed)
- One cup of red onion (chopped)
- Three tbsps. of lime juice
- One-eighth tsp. of black pepper (ground)

**Method:**

1. Mix onion powder, sugar, allspice, thyme, black pepper, salt, cayenne pepper, cloves, and nutmeg in a bowl. Transfer the prepared rub to another bowl and reserve one tbsp. for the pork. Add shredded coconut to the one tbsp. of rub and mix.

2. Preheat your air fryer to 175 degrees Celsius.

3. Start threading the chunks of pork onto the skewers. Use some oil for brushing the pork and then sprinkle the rub on all sides. Place the prepared skewers in the air fryer basket.

4. Cook for eight minutes.

5. Mash one-third of the mango in a bowl and add black beans, lime juice, onion, remaining mango, cilantro, honey, pepper, and salt.

6. Serve the pork skewers with mango mixture by the side.

## Pork Tenderloin With Mustard Crust

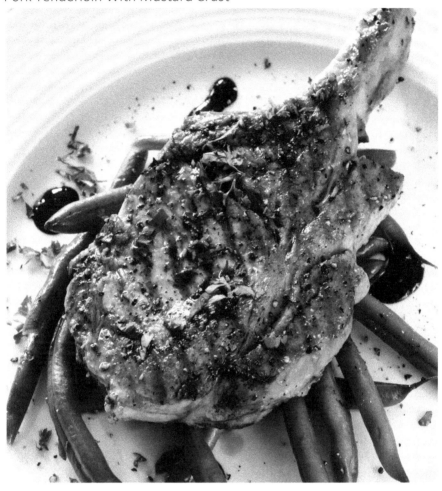

Total Prep & Cooking Time: Forty minutes

Yields: Forty servings

Nutrition Facts: Calories: 280 | Protein: 24.3g | Carbs: 30.2g | Fat: 6.1g | Fiber: 4.9g

**Ingredients**

- One-fourth cup of Dijon mustard
- Two tbsps. of brown sugar
- One tsp. of parsley flakes
- Half tsp. of thyme (dried)
- One-fourth tsp. of each
  - Black pepper (ground)
  - Salt
- Two pounds of pork tenderloin
- One pound of small potatoes
- Twelve ounces of green beans (trimmed)
- One tbsp. of olive oil

**Method:**

1. Start by preheating your air fryer at 200 degrees Celsius.

2. Combine brown sugar, mustard, thyme, parsley, pepper, and salt together in a bowl. Coat the tenderloins with the marinade evenly on all sides.

3. Combine green beans, potatoes, and olive oil in another bowl. Use pepper and salt for seasoning.

4. Cook the pork for twenty minutes. Flip the pork and cook again for five minutes.

5. Let the pork sit for ten minutes.

6. Cook potatoes and green beans for ten minutes in the air fryer.

7. Serve pork with green beans and potatoes by the side.

# Chapter 2: Beef And Fish Recipes

There are various types of beef and fish recipes that can be made using an air fryer. Let's have a look at them.

## Beef Tenderloin

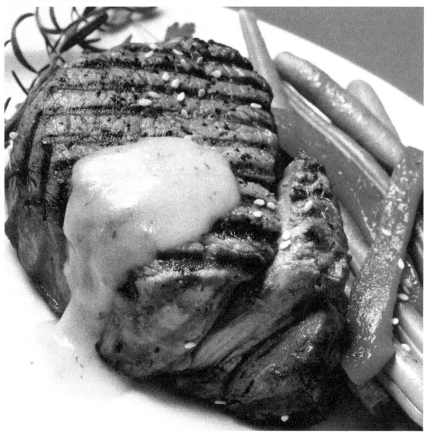

Total Prep & Cooking Time: One hour

Yields: Eight servings

Nutrition Facts: Calories: 230.2 | Protein: 31.2g | Carbs: 0.2g | Fat: 10.3g | Fiber: 0.1g

## Ingredients

- Two pounds of beef tenderloin
- One tbsp. of each
  - Oregano (dried)
  - Vegetable oil
- One tsp. of salt
- Half tsp. of black pepper (cracked)

## Method:

1. Preheat your air fryer at 200 degrees Celsius.

2. Use a paper towel to dry the beef tenderloin.

3. Drizzle some oil over the tenderloin and sprinkle pepper, oregano, and salt. Rub all the spices along with the oil evenly on the meat.

4. Reduce the air fryer heat to 190 degrees Celsius and cook the beef for twenty minutes. Reduce the air fryer heat to 180 degrees Celsius. Cook again for ten minutes.

5. Let the beef rest for ten minutes.

6. Slice the tenderloin and serve warm.

Beef Wontons

Total Prep & Cooking Time: Thirty minutes

Yields: Twenty-four servings

Nutrition Facts: Calories: 73.2 | Protein: 4.4g | Carbs: 5.9g | Fat: 2.6g | Fiber: 0.3g

## Ingredients

- One pound of lean beef (ground)
- Two tbsps. of green onion (chopped)
- Half tsp. of each
    o Garlic powder
    o Salt
- One-fourth tsp. of each
    o Ginger (ground)
    o Black pepper (ground)
- Sixteen ounces of wonton wrappers
- Two tbsps. of sesame oil

## Method:

1. Mix green onions, beef, garlic powder, salt, ginger, and pepper in a large bowl.

2. Preheat your air fryer at 175 degrees Celsius.

3. Place the wrappers on a large plate.

4. Take one tbsp. of the prepared beef mixture and add it to the wonton wrapper. Wet your finger with some water and fold the wrappers in half for forming a triangle.

5. Use sesame oil for brushing each side of the prepared wontons.

6. Cook them in the air fryer for four minutes.

7. Serve hot.

## Mushrooms and Steak

Total Prep & Cooking Time: Four hours and fifty minutes

Yields: Forty servings

Nutrition Facts: Calories: 220 | Protein: 19.1g | Carbs: 5.7g | Fat: 12g | Fiber: 0.7g

### Ingredients

- One pound of beef sirloin steak (cut in cubes of one inch)
- Eight ounces of button mushrooms (sliced)
- One-fourth cup of Worcestershire sauce
- One tbsp. of olive oil
- One tsp. of parsley flakes
- Half tsp. of paprika
- One-third tsp. of chili flakes (crushed)

### Method:

1. Mix mushrooms, steak, olive oil, Worcestershire sauce, paprika, parsley, and chili flakes in a mixing bowl. Refrigerate the mixture for four hours.

2. Take out the mixture thirty minutes prior to your cooking.

3. Preheat your air fryer at a temperature of 200 degrees Celsius.

4. Drain all the marinade. Place the mushrooms and steak into the air fryer basket.

5. Cook for five minutes. Toss the mixture and cook again for five minutes.

Rib Eye Steak

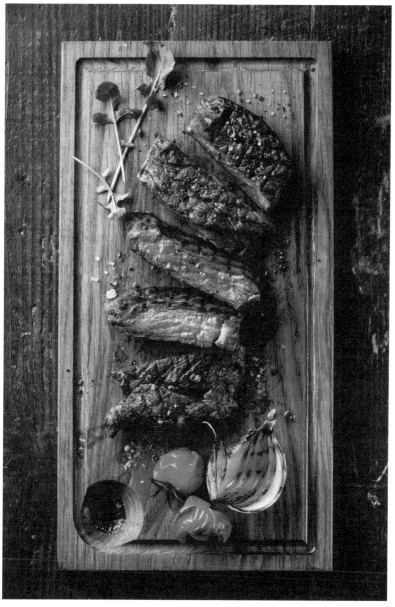

Total Prep & Cooking Time: Two hours and twenty-five minutes

Yields: Two servings

Nutrition Facts: Calories: 650 | Protein: 41.3g | Carbs: 7.2g | Fat: 48.1g | Fiber: 0.9g

**Ingredients**

- Two rib-eye steaks
- Four tsps. of grill seasoning
- One-fourth cup of olive oil
- Half cup soy sauce

**Method:**

1. Mix soy sauce, steak, seasoning, and olive oil in a large bowl. Marinate the steaks for two hours.

2. Add one tbsp. of water to the base of the basket for preventing smoking at the time of cooking.

3. Preheat to 200 degrees Celsius.

4. Add the marinated steaks and cook for seven minutes. Flip the steaks and cook again for seven minutes.

5. Let the steaks it for five minutes.

6. Serve warm.

# Meatloaf

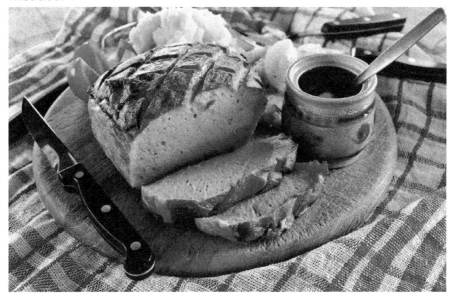

Total Prep & Cooking Time: Forty-five minutes

Yields: Forty servings

Nutrition Facts: Calories: 290 | Protein: 23.8g | Carbs: 5.6g | Fat: 17.6g | Fiber: 0.9g

**Ingredients**

- One pound of lean beef (ground)
- One large egg (beaten)
- Three tbsps. of bread crumbs
- One onion (chopped)

- One tbsp. of thyme (chopped)
- One tsp. of salt
- Half tsp. of black pepper (ground)
- Two mushrooms (sliced thick)
- Half tbsp. of olive oil

**Method:**

1. Start by preheating the air fryer at 200 degrees Celsius.

2. Mix egg, beef, bread crumbs, thyme, onion, pepper, and salt together in a bowl. Mix well.

3. Transfer the mixture of beef to the basket and use a spatula for smoothening the top. Take the mushrooms and press them at the top. Coat the loaf with some olive oil.

4. Set the timer to twenty-five minutes.

5. Let the meatloaf sit for ten minutes.

6. Slice in wedges and serve.

## Fish Sticks

Total Prep & Cooking Time: Twenty minutes

Yields: Forty servings

Nutrition Facts: Calories: 183.2 | Protein: 25.6g | Carbs: 15.2g | Fat: 4.4g | Fiber: 0.9g

**Ingredients**

- One pound of cod fillets
- One-fourth cup of flour
- One large egg
- Half cup of bread crumbs
- One cup of parmesan cheese (grated)
- One tbsp. of parsley flakes
- One tsp. of paprika
- Half tsp. of black pepper (ground)
- One serving of cooking spray

**Method:**

1. Start by preheating your air fryer at 200 degrees Celsius.

2. Use paper towels for pat drying the fillets of fish. Cut the fillets into sticks of half an inch.

3. Add flour in a flat dish.

4. Break the egg and beat in a separate bowl.

5. Combine cheese, bread crumbs, paprika, parsley, and pepper in another dish.

6. Coat the fish sticks in flour and then dip in egg. Coat the sticks with bread crumb mixture.

7. Use a cooking spray for greasing the basket of the air fryer. Arrange the fish stick in the basket.

8. Cook for five minutes. Turn the sticks and cook again for five minutes.

9. Serve hot.

## Cajun Salmon
Total Prep & Cooking Time: Twenty minutes

Yields: Two servings

Nutrition Facts: Calories: 321 | Protein: 31.7g | Carbs: 4.2g | Fat: 17.2g | Fiber: 0.6g

**Ingredients**

- Two fillets of salmon
- One serving of cooking spray
- One tbsp. of Cajun seasoning
- One tsp. of brown sugar

**Method:**

1. Dry the fish fillets using paper towels.

2. Use a cooking spray for misting the fillets.

3. Mix Cajun seasoning along with brown sugar in a bowl. Transfer the mixture into a flat dish.

4. Press the fillets of fish into the mixture of spices.

5. Spray the air fryer basket with cooking spray. Place the fillets with the skin-side down.

6. Cook the fish for eight minutes.

7. Let the fish sit for two minutes.

8. Serve hot.

## Salmon Cakes and Sriracha Mayo
Total Prep & Cooking Time: Forty minutes

Yields: Four servings

Nutrition Facts: Calories: 329 | Protein: 24.3g | Carbs: 3.5g | Fat: 23.2g | Fiber: 2.5g

**Ingredients**

*For sriracha mayo:*

- One tbsp. of sriracha
- One-fourth cup of mayonnaise

*For salmon cakes:*

- One pound fillets of salmon (cut in pieces of one inch)
- One-third cup of almond flour
- One large egg (beaten)
- Two tsps. of seafood seasoning
- One green onion (chopped)
- One serving of cooking spray

**Method:**

1. Mix sriracha and mayonnaise in a bowl. Reserve one tbsp. of the mayo and refrigerate the rest.

2. Add almond flour, salmon, one and a half tsps. of seafood seasoning, egg, reserve sriracha mayo, and green onion to a food processor. Pulse the ingredients for five minutes.

3. Line a dish with parchment paper. Make eight patties from the mixture of fish. Chill the patties in the refrigerator for ten minutes.

4. Preheat your air fryer at 200 degrees Celsius. Use a cooking spray for greasing the basket.

5. Mist the patties with cooking spray and place them in the basket.

6. Cook for eight minutes.

7. Serve the salmon cakes with sriracha mayo by the side.

## Cod With Sesame Crust and Snap Peas

Total Prep & Cooking Time: Thirty minutes

Yields: Four servings

Nutrition Facts: Calories: 356 | Protein: 30.2g | Carbs: 21.3g | Fat: 14.1g | Fiber: 7.2g

**Ingredients**

- Four fillets of cod
- One pinch of black pepper and salt
- Three tbsps. of butter (melted)
- Two tbsps. of sesame seeds
- One tbsp. of vegetable oil
- Two packs of snap peas
- Three garlic cloves (sliced thinly)
- One orange (cut in wedges)

**Method:**

1. Use vegetable oil for brushing the basket of the air fryer. Preheat at 200 degrees Celsius.

2. Sprinkle the fillets of cod with some pepper and salt.

3. Mix sesame seeds and butter in a bowl.

4. Toss garlic and peas with some butter.

5. Cook the peas in the air fryer for ten minutes.

6. Brush the fillets of fish with the mixture of butter and cook for four minutes. Flip the fillets and brush with the remaining butter mixture. Cook again for five minutes.

7. Serve the fish fillets with orange wedges and snap peas.

Grilled Fish and Pesto Sauce

Total Prep & Cooking Time: Twenty minutes

Yields: Two servings

Nutrition Facts: Calories: 1012 | Protein: 44.3g | Carbs: 3.2g | Fat: 93g | Fiber: 2.1g

**Ingredients**

- Two fillets of white fish
- One tsp. of olive oil
- Half tsp. of each
    - Black pepper (ground)
    - Salt

*For the pesto sauce:*

- One bunch of basil
- Two cloves of garlic
- One tbsp. of pine nuts
- Two tbsps. of parmesan cheese (grated)
- One cup of olive oil (extra virgin)

**Method:**

1. Heat your air fryer at 180 degrees Celsius.

2. Brush the fillets of fish with some oil. Sprinkle salt and pepper.

3. Cook the fish fillets for eight minutes.

4. Add garlic, basil leaves, cheese, pine nuts, and olive oil in a blender. Pulse the ingredients until a thick sauce forms.

5. Serve the fish fillets with pesto sauce from the top.

# Chapter 3: Vegetarian Party Recipes

Besides cooking meat in an air fryer, you can also cook various vegetarian dishes with its help. In this section, you will find some tasty vegetarian dishes that you can make with the help of an air fryer.

## Apple Pies
Total Prep & Cooking Time: Forty-five minutes

Yields: Four servings

Nutrition Facts: Calories: 476 | Protein: 3.3g | Carbs: 58.7g | Fat: 27.6g | Fiber: 3.6g

**Ingredients**

- Four tbsps. of butter
- Six tbsps. of brown sugar
- One tsp. of cinnamon (ground)
- Two apples (diced)
- Half tsp. of cornstarch
- Two tsps. of cold water
- Half package of pastry
- One serving of cooking spray

- Half tbsp. of grapeseed oil
- One-fourth cup of powdered sugar
- One tsp. of milk

**Method:**

1. Mix butter, apples, brown sugar, and ground cinnamon in a bowl. Add the mixture to a skillet and cook for five minutes until the apples are soft.

2. Combine cornstarch in water. Add the cornstarch mixture to the skillet.

3. Cook for one minute and keep aside.

4. Unroll the pastry crust and roll it out on a work surface with some flour. Cut the flattened dough in rectangles.

5. Place some apple filling at the center of each rectangle and fold the rectangles for sealing the pie.

6. Use a sharp knife for cutting small slits at the top.

7. Brush some oil at the top and cook for eight minutes at 195 degrees Celsius.

8. Combine milk and sugar in a bowl.

9. Serve the warm pies with sugar glaze from the top.

Fruit Crumble

Total Prep & Cooking Time: Thirty minutes

Yields: Two servings

Nutrition Facts: Calories: 308 | Protein: 2.3g | Carbs: 47.9g | Fat: 7.2g | Fiber: 5.3g

**Ingredients**

- One medium-sized apple
- Half cup of blueberries (frozen)
- One-fourth cup of brown rice flour
- Two tbsps. of sugar
- Half tsp. of cinnamon (ground)
- Three tbsps. of butter

**Method:**

1. Preheat your air fryer for five minutes at 170 degrees Celsius.

2. Mix blueberries and apple in a bowl.

3. Take a bowl and mix sugar, flour, butter, and cinnamon.

4. Pour the mixture of flour over the mixture of fruits.

5. Cook the fruits in the air fryer for fifteen minutes at 170 degrees Celsius.

Kiwi Chips
Total Prep & Cooking Time: One hour

Yields: Six servings

Nutrition Facts: Calories: 110 | Protein: 2.1g | Carbs: 26.3g | Fat: 1.1g | Fiber: 1.3g

**Ingredients**

- One kg of kiwi
- Half tsp. of cinnamon (ground)
- One-fourth tsp. of nutmeg (ground)

**Method:**

1. Slice the kiwi thinly. Keep them in a bowl.

2. Sprinkle nutmeg and cinnamon from the top. Toss for mixing.

3. Preheat the air fryer at 165 degrees Celsius.

4. Cook the kiwi in the air fryer for half an hour. Make sure you shake the basket halfway.

5. Let the chips cool down in the basket for fifteen minutes.

6. Cool before serving.

## Apple Crisp

Total Prep & Cooking Time: Twenty-five minutes

Yields: Two servings

Nutrition Facts: Calories: 341 | Protein: 3.9g | Carbs: 60.5g | Fat: 12.3g | Fiber: 6.9g

**Ingredients**

- Two apples (chopped)
- One tsp. of each
  - Lemon juice
  - Cinnamon
- Two tbsps. of brown sugar

*For the topping:*

- Three tbsps. of flour
- Two tbsps. of brown sugar
- Half tsp. of salt
- Four tbsps. of rolled oats
- One and a half tbsps. of butter

**Method:**

1. Heat your air fryer at 170 degrees Celsius. Use butter for greasing the basket.

2. Combine lemon juice, apples, cinnamon, and sugar together in a bowl.

3. Cook the mixture for fifteen minutes. Shake the basket and cook again for five minutes.

4. For the topping, mix sugar, flour, salt, butter, and oats. Use an electric mixer for mixing.

5. Scatter the topping over the cooked apples.

6. Return the basket to the air fryer. Cook again for five minutes.

Roasted Veggies

Total Prep & Cooking Time: Thirty minutes

Yields: Four servings

Nutrition Facts: Calories: 35 | Protein: 1.3g | Carbs: 3.3g | Fat: 2.6g | Fiber: 1.6g

**Ingredients**

- Half cup of each
    - Summer squash (diced)
    - Zucchini (diced)
    - Mushrooms (diced)
    - Cauliflower (diced)
    - Asparagus (diced)
    - Sweet red pepper (diced)
- Two tsps. of vegetable oil
- One-fourth tsp. of salt
- Half tsp. of black pepper (ground)
- One tsp. of seasoning

**Method:**

1. Preheat air fryer at 180 degrees Celsius.

2. Mix all the veggies, oil, pepper, seasoning, and salt in a bowl. Toss well for coating.

3. Cook the mixture of veggies in the air fryer for ten minutes.

## Tempura Vegetables

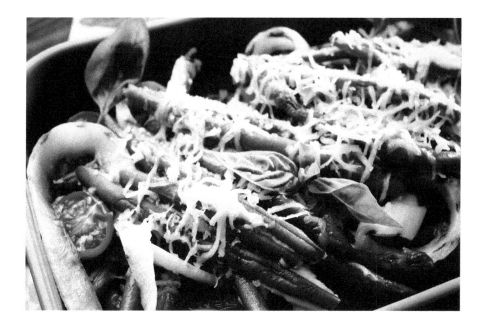

Total Prep & Cooking Time: Thirty-five minutes

Yields: Four servings

Nutrition Facts: Calories: 242 | Protein: 9.2g | Carbs: 35.6g | Fat: 9.3g | Fiber: 3.7g

**Ingredients**

- Half cup of each
  - Flour
  - Green beans
  - Onion rings

- o   Asparagus spears
- o   Sweet pepper rings
- o   Zucchini slices
- o   Avocado wedges
- Half tsp. of each
  - o   Black pepper (ground)
  - o   Salt
- Two large eggs
- Two tbsps. of water
- One cup of panko bread crumbs
- Two tsps. of vegetable oil

**Method:**

1. Combine flour, pepper, and one-fourth tsp. of salt in a dish.

2. Combine water and eggs in a shallow dish.

3. Mix oil and bread crumbs in another shallow dish.

4. Sprinkle remaining salt over the veggies.

5. Dip the veggies in the mixture of flour, then in the mixture of egg, and then coat in bread crumbs.

6. Cook the veggies in the air fryer for ten minutes. Shake in between.

Eggplant Parmesan

Total Prep & Cooking Time: Thirty-five minutes

Yields: Four servings

Nutrition Facts: Calories: 370 | Protein: 24g | Carbs: 35.6g | Fat: 17g | Fiber: 8.6g

**Ingredients**

- Half cup of bread crumbs (Italian)
- One-fourth cup of parmesan cheese (grated)
- One tsp. of each
    o Salt
    o Italian seasoning
- Half tsp. of each
    o Basil (dried)
    o Garlic powder
    o Onion powder
    o Black pepper (ground)
- One cup of flour
- Two large eggs (beaten)
- One eggplant (sliced in round of half an inch)
- One-third cup of marinara sauce
- Eight slices of mozzarella cheese

**Method:**

1. Mix parmesan cheese, bread crumbs, seasoning, basil, salt, onion powder, garlic powder, and black pepper together in a mixing bowl.

2. Add flour in a shallow dish.

3. Beat the eggs in a bowl.

4. Dip the slices of eggplants in flour and then in eggs. Coat the eggplants in the mixture of bread crumbs.

5. Cook the eggplants in the air fryer for ten minutes. Flip and cook for four minutes.

6. Top the slices of eggplants with one slice of mozzarella cheese and marinara sauce.

7. Cook again for two minutes.

8. Serve hot.

## French Fries

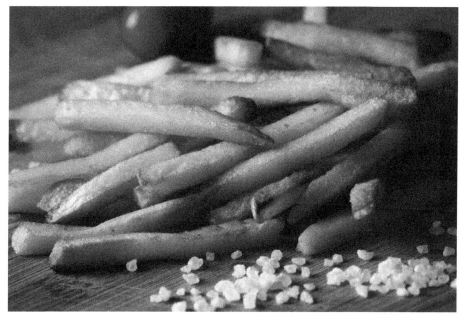

Total Prep & Cooking Time: One hour

Yields: Four servings

Nutrition Facts: Calories: 108 | Protein: 2.4g | Carbs: 17.9g | Fat: 2.1g | Fiber: 3.2g

**Ingredients**

- One pound of russet potatoes (peeled)
- Two tsps. of vegetable oil
- One pinch of cayenne pepper
- Half tsp. of salt

**Method:**

1. Cut the potatoes in half-inch slices lengthwise.

2. Soak the potatoes in water for five minutes.

3. Drain the water and soak again in boiling water for ten minutes.

4. Drain all the water. Pat dry using paper towels.

5. Add oil and cayenne pepper. Season with salt.

6. Cook the potatoes for fifteen minutes. Toss with some salt and cook again for five minutes.

## Sweet and Spicy Carrots

Total Prep & Cooking Time: Thirty minutes

Yields: Two servings

Nutrition Facts: Calories: 128 | Protein: 1.2g | Carbs: 17.2g | Fat: 6g | Fiber: 4.5g

**Ingredients**

- One serving of cooking spray
- One tbsp. of each
  - Hot honey
  - Butter (melted)
  - Orange zest
  - Orange juice
- Half tsp. of cardamom (ground)
- Half pound of baby carrots
- One-third tsp. of black pepper and salt

**Method:**

1. Heat your air fryer at 200 degrees Celsius. Use a cooking spray for greasing the basket.

2. Mix honey, butter, cardamom, and orange zest in a small bowl.

3. Pour the sauce over the carrots and coat well.

4. Cook the carrots for seven twenty minutes. Toss in between.

5. Mix orange juice with the leftover sauce.

6. Serve the carrots with sauce from the top.

## Baked Potatoes

Total Prep & Cooking Time: One hour and five minutes

Yields: Two servings

Nutrition Facts: Calories: 310 | Protein: 7.2g | Carbs: 61.5g | Fat: 6.3g | Fiber: 8.2g

**Ingredients**

- Two large potatoes
- One tbsp. of peanut oil
- Half tsp. of sea salt

**Method:**

1. Heat your air fryer at 200 degrees Celsius.

2. Brush the potatoes with oil. Sprinkle some salt.

3. Place the potatoes in the basket of the air fryer and cook for one hour.

4. Serve hot by dividing the potatoes from the center.

# Chapter 4: Vegetarian Appetizer Recipes

You can prepare various vegetarian appetizer recipes with the help of an air fryer. Let's have a look at them.

## Crunchy Brussels Sprouts

Total Prep & Cooking Time: Fifteen minutes

Yields: Two servings

Nutrition Facts: Calories: 92 | Protein: 5.2g | Carbs: 12.1g | Fat: 3.1g | Fiber: 3.2g

**Ingredients**

- One tsp. of avocado oil
- Half tsp. of each
  - Black pepper (ground)
  - Salt
- Ten ounces of Brussels sprouts (halved)
- One-third tsp. of balsamic vinegar

**Method:**

1. Heat the air fryer at 175 degrees Celsius.

2. Mix salt, pepper, and oil together in a bowl. Add the sprouts and toss.

3. Fry the Brussels sprouts in the air fryer for five minutes.

Buffalo Cauliflower

Total Prep & Cooking Time: Twenty-five minutes

Yields: Four servings

Nutrition Facts: Calories: 190 | Protein: 12.3g | Carbs: 2.3g | Fat: 12g | Fiber: 1.3g

**Ingredients**

- One large cauliflower
- One cup of flour
- One-fourth tsp. of each
  - Chili powder
  - Cayenne pepper
  - Paprika
- One cup of soy milk
- Two tbsps. of butter
- Two garlic cloves (minced)
- Half cup of cayenne pepper sauce
- One serving of cooking spray

**Method:**

1. Cut the cauliflower into small pieces. Rinse under cold water and drain.

2. Mix flour, chili powder, cayenne, and paprika in a bowl. Add the milk slowly for making a thick batter.

3. Add the pieces of cauliflower in the batter and coat well.

4. Cook the cauliflower in the air fryer for twenty minutes. Toss the cauliflower and cook again for ten minutes.

5. Take a saucepan and heat the butter in it. Add garlic and hot sauce. Boil the sauce mixture and simmer for two minutes.

6. Transfer the cauliflower to a large bowl and pour the prepared sauce over the cooked cauliflower. Toss for combining.

7. Serve hot.

## Stuffed Mushrooms

Total Prep & Cooking Time: Thirty minutes

Yields: Six servings

Nutrition Facts: Calories: 42 | Protein: 3.1g | Carbs: 2.9g | Fat: 1.2g | Fiber: 2.3g

## Ingredients

- Fifteen button mushrooms
- One tsp. of olive oil
- One-eighth tsp. of salt
- Half tsp. of black pepper (crushed)
- One-third tsp. of balsamic vinegar

*For the filling:*

- One-fourth cup of each
  - Bell pepper
  - Onion
- Two tbsps. of cilantro (chopped)
- One tbsp. of jalapeno (chopped finely)
- Half cup of mozzarella cheese (grated)
- One tsp. of coriander (ground)
- One-fourth tsp. of each
  - Paprika
  - Salt

**Method:**

1. Use a damp cloth for cleaning the mushrooms. Remove the stems for making the caps hollow.

2. Take a bowl and season the mushroom caps with salt, oil, balsamic vinegar, and black pepper.

3. Take another bowl and mix the ingredients for the filling.

4. Use a spoon for filling the mushroom caps. Press the filling in the mushroom using the backside of the spoon.

5. Cook the mushrooms in the air fryer for ten minutes.

6. Serve hot.

## Sweet Potatoes With Baked Taquitos

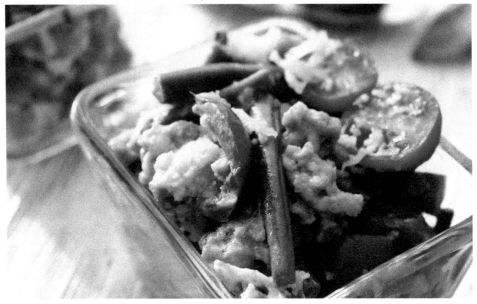

Total Prep & Cooking Time: Forty-five minutes

Yields: Five servings

Nutrition Facts: Calories: 112 | Protein: 5.2g | Carbs: 19.3g | Fat: 1.6g | Fiber: 6.1g

**Ingredients**

- One sweet potato (cut in pieces of half an inch)
- Two tsps. of canola oil
- Half cup yellow onion (chopped)
- One garlic clove (minced)
- Two cups of black beans (rinsed)
- One chipotle pepper (chopped)

- Half tsp. of each
  - Paprika
  - Cumin
  - Chili powder
  - Maple syrup
- One-eighth tsp. of salt
- Three tbsps. of water
- Ten corn tortillas

## Method:

1. Place the pieces of sweet potatoes in an air fryer and toss it with some oil. Cook for twelve minutes. Make sure you shake the basket in between.

2. Take a skillet and heat some oil in it. Add the garlic and onions. Sauté for five minutes until the onions are translucent.

3. Add chipotle pepper, beans, paprika, cumin, chili powder, maple syrup, and salt. Add two tbsps. of water and mix all the ingredients.

4. Add cooked potatoes and mix well.

5. Warm the corn tortillas in a skillet.

6. Put two tbsps. of beans and potato mixture in a row across the corn tortillas. Grab one end of the corn tortillas and roll them. Tuck the end under the mixture of sweet potato and beans.

7. Place the taquitos with the seam side down in the basket. Spray the taquitos with some oil. Air fry the prepared taquitos for ten minutes.

8. Serve hot.

## Cauliflower Curry

Total Prep & Cooking Time: Twenty minutes

Yields: Three servings

Nutrition Facts: Calories: 160 | Protein: 5.2g | Carbs: 27.2g | Fat: 3.1g | Fiber: 5.6g

### Ingredients

- One cup of vegetable stock
- Three-fourth cup of coconut milk (light)
- Two tsps. of curry powder
- One tsp. of garlic puree
- Half tsp. of turmeric
- Twelve ounces of cauliflower (cut in florets)
- One and a half cup of sweet corn kernels
- Three spring onions (sliced)
- Salt

*For the topping:*

- Lime wedges
- Two tbsps. of dried cranberries

### Method:

1. Heat your air fryer at 190 degrees Celsius.

2. Mix all ingredients in a large bowl. Combine well.

3. Transfer the cauliflower mixture to the air fryer basket.

4. Cook for fifteen minutes. Give it a mix in the middle.

## Air-Fried Avocado Wedges

Total Prep & Cooking Time: Twenty minutes

Yields: Two servings

Nutrition Facts: Calories: 302 | Protein: 8.3g | Carbs: 37.2g | Fat: 17.3g | Fiber: 7.4g

### Ingredients

- One-fourth cup of flour
- Half tsp. of black pepper (ground)
- One-fourth tsp. of salt
- One tsp. of water
- One ripe avocado (cut in eight slices)
- Half cup of bread crumbs
- One serving of cooking spray

### Method:

1. Heat your air fryer at 200 degrees Celsius.

2. Combine pepper, salt, and flour in a bowl. Place water in another bowl.

3. Take a shallow dish and spread the bread crumbs.

4. Coat the avocado slices in flour mixture and dip it in water.

5. Coat the slices in bread crumbs. Make sure both sides are evenly coated.

6. Use cooking spray for misting the slices of avocado.

7. Cook the coated slices of avocado for four minutes. Flip the slices and cook again for three minutes.

8. Serve hot.

Crunchy Grains

Total Prep & Cooking Time: Twenty minutes

Yields: Four servings

Nutrition Facts: Calories: 71 | Protein: 5.8g | Carbs: 34.4g | Fat: 3.2g | Fiber: 7.3g

**Ingredients**

- Three cups of whole grains (cooked)
- Half cup of peanut oil

**Method:**

1. Use a paper towel for removing excess moisture from the grains.

2. Toss the grains in oil.

3. Add the coated grains in the basket of the air fryer. Cook for ten minutes. Toss the grains and cook again for five minutes.

## Buffalo Chickpeas

Total Prep & Cooking Time: Thirty minutes

Yields: Two servings

Nutrition Facts: Calories: 172 | Protein: 7.2g | Carbs: 31.6g | Fat: 1.4g | Fiber: 7.4g

**Ingredients**

- One can of chickpeas (rinsed)
- Two tbsps. of buffalo wing sauce
- One tbsp. of ranch dressing mix (dry)

**Method:**

1. Heat your air fryer at 175 degrees Celsius.

2. Use paper towels for removing excess moisture from the chickpeas.

3. Transfer the chickpeas to a bowl and add the wing sauce. Add the dressing mix and combine well.

4. Cook the chickpeas in the air fryer for eight minutes. Shake the basket and cook for five minutes.

5. Let the chickpeas sit for two minutes.

6. Serve warm.

Easy Falafel

Total Prep & Cooking Time: Forty minutes

Yields: Fifteen servings

Nutrition Facts: Calories: 57.9 | Protein: 3.2g | Carbs: 8.9g | Fat: 1.4g | Fiber: 3.9g

**Ingredients**

- One cup of garbanzo beans
- Two cups of cilantro (remove the stems)
- Three-fourth cup of parsley (remove the stems)
- On red onion (quartered)
- One garlic clove
- Two tbsps. of chickpea flour
- One tbsp. of each
  - Cumin (ground)
  - Coriander (ground)
  - Sriracha sauce
- One tsp. of black pepper and salt (for seasoning)
- Half tsp. of each
  - Baking soda
  - Baking powder
- One serving of cooking spray

**Method:**

1. Soak the beans in cool water for one day. Rub the beans and remove the skin. Rinse in cold water and use paper towels for removing excess moisture.

2. Add cilantro, beans, onion, parsley, and garlic in a blender. Blend the ingredients until paste forms.

3. Transfer the blended paste to a bowl and add coriander, flour, sriracha, cumin, pepper, and salt. Mix well. Let the mixture sit for twenty minutes.

4. Add baking soda and baking powder to the mixture. Mix well.

5. Make fifteen balls from the mixture and flatten them using your hands for making patties.

6. Usea cooking spray for greasing the falafel patties.

7. Cook them for ten minutes.

8. Serve warm.

Mini Cheese and Bean Tacos

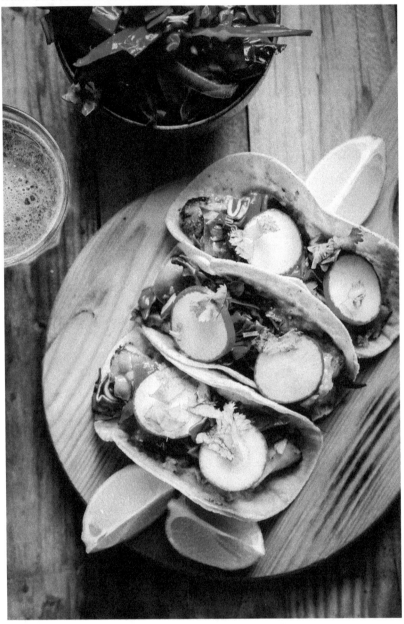

Total Prep & Cooking Time: Thirty minutes

Yields: Twelve servings

Nutrition Facts: Calories: 229 | Protein: 11.3g | Carbs: 20.2g | Fat: 10.4g | Fiber: 2.9g

**Ingredients**

- One can of refried beans
- One ounce of taco seasoning mix
- Twelve slices of American cheese (halved)
- Twelve tortillas
- One serving of cooking spray

**Method:**

1. Place the beans in a medium-sized bowl. Add the seasoning mix. Combine well.

2. Place one cheese piece in the center of each tortilla. Take one tbsp. of the bean mix and add it over the cheese. Add another cheese piece over the beans. Fold the tortillas in half. Gently press with your hands for sealing the ends.

3. Use cooking spray for spraying the tacos.

4. Cook the tacos for three minutes. Turn the tacos and cook again for three minutes

5. Serve hot.

## Green Beans and Spicy Sauce

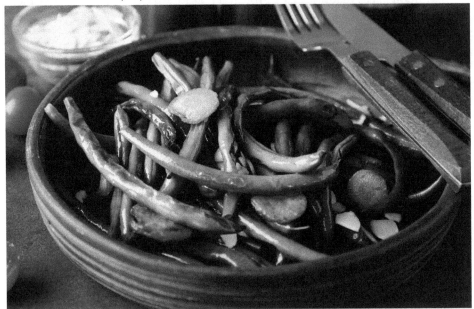

Total Prep & Cooking Time: Thirty minutes

Yields: Four servings

Nutrition Facts: Calories: 460.2 | Protein: 5.7g | Carbs: 34.4g | Fat: 30.6g | Fiber: 4.2g

**Ingredients**

- One cup of beer
- One and a half cup of flour
- Two tsps. of salt
- Half tsp. of black pepper (ground)
- Twelve ounces of green beans (trimmed)

*For the sauce:*

- One cup of ranch dressing
- Two tsps. of sriracha sauce
- One tsp. of horseradish

**Method:**

1. Mix flour, beer, pepper, and salt in a mixing bowl. Add the beans in the batter and coat well. Shake off extra batter.

2. Line the air fryer basket with parchment paper. Add the beans and cook for ten minutes. Shake in between.

3. Combine sriracha sauce, ranch dressing, and horseradish together in a bowl.

4. Serve the beans with sauce by the side.

Cheesy Sugar Snap Peas
Total Prep & Cooking Time: Fifteen minutes

Yields: Four servings

Nutrition Facts: Calories: 72 | Protein: 5.7g | Carbs: 8.9g | Fat: 3.3g | Fiber: 2.5g

## Ingredients

- Half pound of sugar snap peas
- One tsp. of olive oil
- One-fourth cup of bread crumbs
- Half cup of parmesan cheese
- Pepper and salt (for seasoning)
- Two tbsps. of garlic (minced)

## Method:

1. Remove the stem from each pea pod. Rinse the peas and drain the water.

2. Toss the peas with bread crumbs, olive oil, pepper, salt, and half of the cheese.

3. Cook the peas in the air fryer for four minutes at 175 degrees Celsius.

4. Add minced garlic and cook again for five minutes.

5. Serve the peas with remaining cheese from the top.